DASH DIET COOKBOOK FOR BEGINNER

Quick, Healthy and Simple Recipes for Everyday Wellness. Low-Sodium Cooking, Delicious and Nutritious | Include 14 Days Meal Plan | New Edition

Iona Kameron

2

TABLE OF CONTENTS

6. Dinners: Simple and Satisfying   **55**

7. Snacks and Sides   **67**

8. Desserts and Treats   **77**

1. INTRODUCTION TO THE DASH DIET

Welcome to a journey that promises not just a transformation of your plate, but a refreshing new perspective on what it means to live healthily. The DASH diet, an acronym that stands for Dietary Approaches to Stop Hypertension, is often celebrated for its practical approach to reducing sodium intake and increasing nutrient-rich foods. Yet, it's so much more than a simple guideline to lower blood pressure—it's about crafting a balanced lifestyle that enhances your overall well-being.

Imagine you're setting the stage for a healthier life where every meal is a step towards renewed vitality. The DASH diet is rooted in a philosophy that embraces whole grains, vegetables, fruits, and lean proteins, while moderating sweets and saturated fats. It's not about stringent restrictions or feeling deprived, but about finding joy in the wholesome flavor's nature offers.

This approach is especially empowering for beginners who might feel overwhelmed by the myriad of dietary trends flooding our feeds. Unlike regimes that require radical changes overnight, the DASH diet is a gentle invitation to make sustainable adjustments. It encourages you to experiment with spices to replace salt, to choose whole foods over processed options, and to appreciate the natural sweetness of fruits instead of reaching for sugary treats.

Here's the beauty of it: every choice is guided by a desire not just to eat, but to nourish and flourish. With each chapter of this book, you'll find yourself more equipped to make informed decisions about what goes on your plate. From understanding the impact of sodium on your body to recognizing the power of a balanced meal, you are taking control of your health—one delicious bite at a time.

As we delve deeper into the principles of the DASH diet, remember that this is not just about avoiding hypertension or maintaining a healthy weight. It's about setting the foundation for a vibrant, energetic life where food is both the pleasure and the remedy. Let this be your guide to exploring new tastes, to rediscovering the joy of cooking, and to cultivating a diet that feels as good as it tastes. Welcome aboard!

UNDERSTANDING THE DASH DIET

Imagine yourself walking through a bustling farmer's market. Each stand bursts with the season's best produce—crisp greens, vibrant berries, and fresh fish caught that morning. As you wander through, you're not just shopping; you're curating the ingredients for your health. This scene captures the essence of the DASH diet, a way of eating that emphasizes the natural, the fresh, and the nutrient-rich.

The DASH diet isn't a fleeting trend but a research-backed approach to eating that holds the power to transform your health. Initially developed in the early 1990s through a series of studies funded by the U.S. National Institutes of Health, the primary goal was straightforward: investigate ways to naturally reduce blood pressure. The results were nothing short of revelatory, showing that a diet low in sodium and rich in fruits, vegetables, whole grains, and lean proteins could significantly lower blood pressure in just a few weeks.

But what exactly does it mean to follow the DASH diet? At its core, it's about balance and making informed choices. It involves a hearty intake of vegetables and fruits, coupled with enough whole grains to keep you full and satisfied. Lean proteins from fish, poultry, and legumes, along with healthy fats from nuts, seeds, and oils, are also key components. Dairy is included too, preferably low-fat or non-fat, providing calcium without excessive saturated fat. And importantly, the diet suggests sweets and red meats be enjoyed sparingly—not eliminated, just lessened.

Let's delve a bit deeper into the mechanics of why this diet works. High blood pressure, or hypertension, is often linked to high sodium intake. The standard American diet is rife with hidden salt, primarily through processed foods. The DASH diet's lower sodium limits help to mitigate this risk, but there's more to it than just cutting out salt. The increase in fruits and vegetables boosts potassium intake, a mineral that supports heart health by helping to balance sodium levels within the body and easing tension in blood vessel walls.

Moreover, this diet naturally increases your intake of dietary fiber, which is found abundantly in whole grains and fresh produce. Fiber not only helps in regulating digestion and keeping you feeling full but also plays a role in managing blood sugar levels and lowering cholesterol. The inclusion of nuts, seeds, and legumes provides additional heart-healthy fats that can help improve cholesterol profiles and enrich the body with essential nutrients like magnesium and zinc.

Understanding the DASH diet also means recognizing what it is not. It's not about rigorous calorie counting or feeling deprived. It's not a commercial diet plan that requires purchasing specialized foods. Instead, it's about embracing food as a pleasurable and powerful way to enhance health. It's about making choices that feel good, taste good, and are good for you.

Consider how empowering it can feel to cook a meal that aligns with such principles. You're not just following recipes; you're crafting a lifestyle that wards off chronic diseases, energizes your body, and calms your mind. The psychological benefits of eating well—knowing that you are nurturing your body with every bite—are profound. Food becomes more than sustenance; it becomes a source of pleasure and a foundation for good health.

Adopting the DASH diet can seem challenging at first, especially if you're accustomed to eating lots of processed foods or if your life is tightly intertwined with the fast-paced conveniences of modern dining. But the transition can be smooth and enjoyable with a focus on incremental change. Start with simple swaps, like choosing whole-grain bread instead of white or integrating a vegetable side into every meal. Each small choice builds upon the last, gradually constructing a healthier dietary pattern that can last a lifetime.

People from various dietary backgrounds and preferences can adapt the DASH diet to fit their needs. Whether you are a vegetarian looking to enhance your meal planning or someone managing diabetes and needing to stabilize blood sugar, the foundational principles of DASH provide a flexible framework that can accommodate a diverse array of nutritional needs. This adaptability not only makes it sustainable over the long term but also inclusive enough to be adopted by nearly anyone, anywhere.

Embracing the DASH diet is like turning each meal into a small celebration of your health. It's a commitment to nourishing your body and enjoying the abundance of benefits that come from thoughtful, intentional eating. It's a pathway paved not just with good intentions, but with delicious, life-enriching food.

BENEFITS OF LOW-SODIUM EATING

Stepping into the world of low-sodium eating is like opening a door to a new dimension of health benefits, one that goes beyond the common notion that it's merely about avoiding salt. Understanding the wide-ranging advantages of reducing sodium in our diet offers a fresh perspective on how we can nurture our bodies and enhance our wellbeing.

For many, the first benefit of cutting back on sodium is the most immediate and motivating: managing blood pressure. When sodium intake decreases, blood pressure often follows suit, reducing the strain on your cardiovascular system. But the positive changes don't stop there. This decrease in pressure can lead to a cascade of benefits, supporting not just the heart but the entire vascular system. Over time, those who maintain a low-sodium diet experience a marked decrease in the risk of cardiovascular diseases, including heart attack and stroke. This is because high blood pressure is a significant risk factor for these conditions, and managing it effectively can lead to longer, healthier lives.

But the advantages extend even further into aspects of health that might not be as obvious. For instance, kidneys, the body's natural filtration system, are highly sensitive to the amount of sodium in the blood. High sodium levels can increase the workload on these organs, potentially leading to damage over time. By adopting a low-sodium lifestyle, you help your kidneys operate more efficiently and reduce the risk of kidney disease. This aspect of dietary sodium is especially crucial for individuals with existing kidney issues, as managing sodium intake can be a key factor in controlling disease progression.

Moreover, a low-sodium diet often correlates with lower rates of osteoporosis. Excessive sodium can cause calcium loss through urine, which in turn weakens bones, making them more susceptible to fractures. By keeping sodium consumption in check, you can help preserve your bone density and ensure a stronger skeletal structure as you age.

Beyond the physical health benefits, the implications for mental wellbeing are equally compelling. High blood pressure can affect cerebral health in several ways, potentially impairing cognitive function. Studies have indicated that individuals on low-sodium diets might have a lower risk of cognitive decline as they age, linked to better overall vascular health and blood pressure management.

The reduction in sodium also often encourages a dietary shift towards whole foods and away from processed options, which are typically high in sodium. This transition can lead to an increased intake of vitamins and minerals that are abundant in fruits, vegetables, and whole grains. The nutritional richness of these foods supports a multitude of bodily functions, from immune defense to energy metabolism, contributing to an overall sense of vitality and wellness.

Imagine a typical day with a low-sodium diet: starting with a breakfast rich in whole grains and fresh fruits, enjoying a lunch loaded with leafy greens and lean proteins, and ending with a dinner that features a bounty of vegetables. Each meal not only delights the palate but also delivers a powerful dose of nutrition, all while keeping your sodium intake in check.

For those who might worry about the flavor sacrifices associated with reducing salt, the culinary creativity that often blossoms from this challenge can be an unexpected benefit. Discovering the natural flavors of foods without the mask of excessive salt can be a revelation. Herbs, spices, and the simple joy of tasting the real essence of fresh ingredients can elevate your cooking, turning meals into a celebration of natural tastes.

Adopting a low-sodium diet does not mean stepping into a world of bland and uninspiring meals. It's about redefining what flavor means, exploring new ingredients, and rediscovering the joy of cooking and eating in a way that nourishes your body and soul. This change can also foster a sense of community as you share your discoveries and recipes with friends and family, spreading the health benefits further.

Lastly, the empowerment that comes from taking control of your diet and, by extension, your health, cannot be underestimated. Learning to manage sodium intake equips you with skills that translate into broader aspects of life management, promoting a proactive attitude towards health that can inspire every choice you make.

Embracing a low-sodium diet is not merely about cutting out salt, but about enhancing the quality of your life, one meal at a time. It's a testament to the fact that the best changes often come with a multitude of rewards, influencing more than just one aspect of our health but enriching our entire life experience.

How This Book Will Guide You

Embarking on a journey toward healthier eating can often feel like setting sail into unknown waters—exciting yet slightly daunting. This book is your compass, designed to navigate the rich and rewarding world of the DASH diet. It's not just about what to eat or what to avoid; it's about understanding the whys and how's of making choices that enhance your well-being. Here's how this guide will support you in embracing a low-sodium, nutritious lifestyle that aligns with your health goals and taste preferences.

From the outset, this book lays a solid foundation of knowledge, exploring the scientific underpinnings of the DASH diet. Understanding why certain foods influence your blood pressure and heart health empowers you to make informed decisions. It's not simply a list of dos and don'ts; it's a deep dive into how your body processes different nutrients and how you can harness this knowledge for your health. Each chapter builds on this foundation, ensuring you know the reasons behind the recommendations.

As you turn the pages, you'll find that this book is structured to gradually introduce you to all aspects of the DASH diet—from the basics of starting a low-sodium diet to sophisticated strategies for maintaining these healthy habits in the long term. It begins with simple, practical steps, ensuring you feel confident before moving on to more advanced concepts. This gradual approach helps to prevent the feeling of being overwhelmed and makes the transition smoother and more manageable.

One of the core features of this guide is its practical application of the DASH diet principles. It offers a realistic, adaptable approach to dieting that considers the challenges of everyday life. Whether you're a busy professional, a parent juggling multiple responsibilities, or someone who's simply trying to make better dietary choices, this book provides strategies that can be tailored to fit your lifestyle. It recognizes that life is not one-size-fits-all and neither is dieting.

To enhance your learning experience, each section is accompanied by illustrative examples and anecdotes from real-life situations. These stories not only provide practical applications of the principles discussed but also make the journey relatable and engaging. They serve as reminders that many others have successfully walked this path and have overcome similar challenges. This narrative approach helps to weave a thread of camaraderie and support throughout the book.

Moreover, this guide doesn't stop at what you eat—it extends to how you prepare your meals. It embraces the joy of cooking by providing tips on how to creatively adapt your favorite dishes to fit the DASH guidelines. The aim is to show that healthy eating does not mean sacrificing flavor or satisfaction. It's about enhancing dishes in ways that boost their nutritional value while still delighting your taste buds.

Acknowledging that change is a process, this book also equips you with tools to track your progress and stay motivated. It introduces simple yet effective ways to monitor your dietary habits and blood pressure, helping you see the tangible benefits of your efforts. This feedback loop is crucial for maintaining motivation, as it allows you to witness the direct impact of your dietary choices on your health.

In addition to nutritional guidance, the book provides insights into how to sustainably integrate the DASH diet into your lifestyle. It includes tips on meal planning, grocery shopping, and dining out, making it easier to stick to your goals even when life gets busy. By anticipating common pitfalls and offering solutions, the book prepares you for long-term success.

Finally, this guide understands that education is a continuous journey. It encourages ongoing learning and provides resources for further exploration, ensuring that you can continue to grow and adapt your approach as new research emerges and as your needs change. It promotes a proactive attitude towards health—a commitment to continually investing in your well-being.

This book is more than just a manual; it's a companion on your journey to better health. It's here to guide, educate, and inspire you as you make the transition to a healthier lifestyle. With each page, you'll gain more than just knowledge; you'll build the confidence to create lasting changes that resonate not just through your diet, but through every aspect of your life.

2. The Basics of Healthy Eating

Embarking on a journey of healthy eating is much like learning a new language. It opens up a world of flavors, gives us new tools to express our care for our bodies, and often, it starts with understanding the basics. This chapter is dedicated to laying down those foundational elements of nutrition that will not only feed your body but also enrich your life.

Healthy eating is often shrouded in complex dietary advice, quick-fix diets, and a maze of do's and don'ts that can seem overwhelming. Here, we strip it back to the essentials. It's about more than just choosing an apple over a bag of chips; it's understanding why that choice might help you feel more vibrant, more energetic, and more balanced.

We'll explore what it means to truly nourish yourself—considering not just the calories but the quality of the foods you eat. This isn't about restrictive eating or unrealistically banning certain foods. Instead, it's about creating a harmonious diet that includes a wide variety of nutrients that support different bodily functions, contribute to your overall health, and help you maintain energy throughout the day.

Throughout this chapter, we'll weave through the practicalities of balancing macronutrients—carbohydrates, proteins, and fats—while highlighting the unsung heroes of our plates: vitamins and minerals. These are the components that often don't get enough attention but have substantial roles in everything from bone health to brain function.

By the end of this chapter, the hope is that you'll view every meal as an opportunity to not only satisfy your hunger but to also care for the most precious home you'll ever have—your body. Let's demystify nutrition and rediscover the joy of eating in ways that feel good, taste good, and are inherently good for you. This is where you start to build a lasting, loving relationship with your food and your health.

Nutritional Foundations

Understanding the nutritional foundations of a healthy diet is akin to building a strong, resilient structure. Just as a house needs a solid base to withstand the elements, our bodies require a diverse range of nutrients to thrive. This chapter will delve into the core components of nutrition—macronutrients and micronutrients—explaining their roles and how they interact to support our health.

Macronutrients: The Big Three

Macronutrients are the nutrients we need in larger amounts, serving as the primary building blocks and fuel sources for our bodies. They include carbohydrates, proteins, and fats, each playing unique and essential roles.

Carbohydrates are often vilified in trendy diet circles, but they are our body's main energy source. They are not just about giving us quick energy boosts; they are crucial for brain function, kidney operation, and muscle activity. The key is to choose complex carbohydrates found in whole grains, fruits, and vegetables, which provide a steady release of energy, thanks to their high fiber content, rather than the quick spikes from sugary snacks.

Proteins are the building blocks of muscle, skin, enzymes, and hormones. They are vital for muscle repair, growth, and overall cellular health. Our bodies require different types of amino acids, some of which are known as essential amino acids because they need to be ingested; our bodies can't produce them. High-quality proteins, which contain all the essential amino acids, are typically found in animal products, though combining various plant-based proteins can also fulfill these needs.

Fats, once unfairly shunned, are now recognized as fundamentally important to our diets. They are crucial for long-term energy, insulation, and cell structure. Fats also aid in the absorption of fat-soluble vitamins (A, D, E, K) and provide essential fatty acids necessary for brain health and controlling inflammation. The focus should be on unsaturated fats, such as those from fish, nuts, seeds, and certain oils, which support heart health.

Micronutrients: Vital Vitamins and Minerals

While we need them in smaller amounts, vitamins and minerals are essential to many bodily functions, from bone health to blood clotting to immune system support. They are crucial for turning the food we eat into energy and repairing cellular damage.

Vitamins are organic compounds that are generally classified into water-soluble and fat-soluble categories. Water-soluble vitamins, like C and all the B-vitamins, must be consumed regularly because they are not stored in the body. Fat-soluble vitamins, such as A, D, E, and K, are stored in the liver and fat tissues, with functions ranging from maintaining vision to protecting the body from antioxidative damage.

Minerals include calcium, potassium, sodium, and iron, playing roles in everything from maintaining healthy bones and teeth to facilitating nerve transmissions and forming hemoglobin, which carries oxygen in the blood.

Balancing Nutrients for Optimal Health

The art of healthy eating is about balancing these nutrients in ways that support your body's needs. The precise balance can vary based on age, sex, activity level, and health goals, but there are general principles that apply universally:

1. **Aim for Variety**: Consuming a wide range of foods ensures a broader intake of nutrients. This means colorful fruits and vegetables, diverse protein sources (both animal and plant-based), and various whole grains.

2. **Mind Your Portions**: Understanding portion sizes helps manage calorie intake and can prevent nutrient imbalances. For instance, a serving of meat should be about the size of a deck of cards, while a serving of cooked pasta should be about a half-cup.

3. **Listen to Your Body**: Paying attention to how foods affect your energy levels, mood, and general health can help tailor your diet more effectively. Foods that consistently make you feel sluggish or irritable should be consumed less frequently or not at all.

Connecting with Food

Our relationship with food is deeply personal and shaped by culture, family traditions, and personal preferences. Recognizing this connection can enhance your appreciation for nutrition and inspire you to make healthier choices that are not only good for the body but also satisfying and culturally significant.

Eating well is an act of self-respect. It says, 'I value my body enough to give it what it needs to thrive.' As you become more familiar with the basics of nutrition, you'll be better equipped to build that sturdy, nourishing structure of a well-balanced diet that sustains you physically, emotionally, and socially. This foundation doesn't just support a healthy body; it supports a vibrant, energetic life.

UNDERSTANDING SODIUM IN YOUR DIET

Sodium is a mineral that's essential for life. It's needed to regulate blood pressure, maintain fluid balance, and support nerve and muscle function. Yet, in the narrative of modern health, sodium often plays the villain, primarily due to its role in high blood pressure and heart disease when consumed in excess. Understanding sodium in your diet is not about casting it out—it's about learning how to use it wisely.

For most of us, sodium consumption is predominantly linked to table salt, which is sodium chloride. However, sodium is also present in various other forms and is hidden in many of the foods we consume daily, especially processed foods. The journey to understanding and managing sodium intake effectively is much like learning to find a balance on a seesaw. It's about achieving the right equilibrium that supports your body without tipping into health risks.

The Role of Sodium in the Body

At a physiological level, sodium is a crucial player. It helps conduct nerve impulses, contracts and relaxes muscles, and maintains the proper balance of water and minerals in the body. It's so vital that the body has a sophisticated system to control blood levels under a tight range. Kidneys adjust the excretion of sodium based on dietary intake; however, when consumption is too high, this system is strained, and sodium starts to accumulate in the blood. Since sodium attracts and holds water, its increased blood concentration leads to higher blood volume, making the heart work harder and increasing pressure in the arteries.

The Consequences of Excessive Sodium

While the body needs sodium, too much can lead to hypertension (high blood pressure), which is a major risk factor for heart disease and stroke, two of the leading causes of death worldwide. But the impact doesn't stop at cardiovascular health. High sodium intake has also been linked to other conditions, such as kidney disease, osteoporosis, and stomach cancer.

Current Dietary Guidelines

Health organizations globally recommend reducing sodium intake to moderate levels. The American Heart Association suggests no more than 2,300 milligrams a day for healthy adults, which is about one teaspoon of table salt, and an ideal limit of no more than 1,500 milligrams per day for most adults, especially those with hypertension. Despite these guidelines, the average intake in many populations remains significantly higher, often because of hidden salts in processed and restaurant foods.

Recognizing and Reducing Sodium Intake

Understanding where sodium lurks in your diet is the first step towards control. Surprisingly, more than 70% of the sodium in a typical diet comes from processed and prepared foods, not from salt added during cooking or at the table. Foods like pizzas, breads, soups, and processed meats are major contributors. The sodium in these foods is not just for taste; it also serves as a preservative and texturizer.

Reducing sodium intake doesn't require a radical diet overhaul. Start with reading labels carefully; food labels are your best tool in identifying high-sodium products. Opt for "low sodium" or "no salt added" versions of staples like canned vegetables, beans, and sauces. When eating out, it can be beneficial to ask how food is prepared and request dishes with no or minimal salt.

Substituting and Savoring

Reducing sodium doesn't mean eating bland food. It's an opportunity to discover the rich flavors of natural foods and experiment with herbs, spices, and citrus to enhance taste without adding extra sodium. Foods rich in potassium, such as bananas, potatoes, and spinach, can also help balance sodium levels in the body.

Monitoring and Adapting

Understanding your own body's response to sodium is crucial. Some people are more sensitive to sodium than others, meaning even small amounts can significantly impact blood pressure. Monitoring your blood pressure as you make dietary changes can help you understand how sensitive you are to sodium. This personal insight allows for a tailored approach to sodium in your diet, which can be more effective than following general guidelines alone.

A Lifelong Balance

Ultimately, managing sodium intake is about creating a balanced diet that supports your long-term health and wellbeing. It's about making informed choices that consider both the pleasures of taste and the necessity of good health. By understanding and adjusting the role of sodium in your diet, you open the door to a healthier life, where food continues to bring joy and nourishment in equal measure.

BALANCING YOUR MEALS

Imagine sitting down to a meal that not only delights your taste buds but also perfectly fulfills your body's nutritional needs. This isn't just a dream for the health-conscious; it's an achievable reality with a little knowledge and preparation. Balancing your meals is about more than just mixing different foods on a plate; it's about combining ingredients in a way that harmonizes your body's nutritional requirements and your personal tastes. This chapter explores how to achieve that balance, ensuring every meal contributes positively to your overall health.

The Art of Meal Composition

Creating a balanced meal begins with understanding the roles that different foods play in our diets. Each food group provides unique nutrients that our bodies need to function optimally. By incorporating a variety of food groups in our meals, we ensure a more complete nutrient profile, which includes macronutrients—proteins, fats, and carbohydrates—as well as essential vitamins and minerals.

Proteins: Building and Repairing

Proteins are fundamental for building and repairing tissues, making enzymes and hormones, and supporting immune function. Including a protein source at each meal helps stabilize blood sugar levels and sustain satiety. Sources can vary widely from meats and fish to legumes and dairy.

Carbohydrates: Energizing the Body

Carbohydrates are the body's main energy source. They break down into glucose, which fuels brain function and physical activity. However, the type of carbohydrates matters. Whole grains, vegetables, and fruits provide not only energy but also important dietary fiber and nutrients, in contrast to the quick highs and rapid lows of refined sugars.

Fats: Supporting Cell Function

Fats have received a bad rap, but they're essential for supporting cell growth, protecting organs, and aiding in nutrient absorption. The key is to choose healthy fats, such as those found in avocados, nuts, seeds, and certain oils, which contribute to cardiovascular health and reduce inflammation.

Understanding Portion Sizes

An essential aspect of balancing meals is understanding portion sizes. Overeating, even of the healthiest foods, can lead to imbalances and health issues. Visual cues can be helpful: a serving of protein should be about the size of your palm, a serving of carbohydrates about the size of your fist, and a serving of fat about the size of your thumb.

The Role of Micronutrients

While macronutrients provide the bulk of dietary energy, micronutrients (vitamins and minerals) play critical roles in ensuring health and vitality. They are crucial for preventing disease and essential for healthy growth and development. Each meal should include a variety of colorful fruits and vegetables to ensure a good mix of micronutrients.

Timing and Frequency of Meals

Balancing your meals also includes considering the timing and frequency of eating. Eating at regular intervals helps maintain energy levels throughout the day and prevents overeating. For some, three meals a day works well, while others may prefer smaller, more frequent meals. Listening to your body's cues and adjusting your eating schedule can help maintain a steady metabolism.

Integrating Diversity on Your Plate

One of the joys of balanced eating is the variety it can introduce to your diet. Each meal offers an opportunity to explore new flavors and cuisines. Diversity in your diet not only makes meals more interesting but also exposes you to a broader range of nutrients. Experiment with different grains, try new fruits and vegetables, and incorporate a variety of protein sources to make each meal both nutritious and exciting.

Managing Special Dietary Needs

Balancing meals becomes slightly more complex when considering food allergies, sensitivities, or specific dietary requirements such as vegetarian or ketogenic diets. However, the principles of balance, diversity, and portion control remain the same. It's about making adjustments within the framework of your dietary needs to ensure that meals are still nutritionally complete.

Practical Tips for Daily Eating

1. **Plan Ahead**: Planning meals can help you maintain balance in your diet. It prevents last-minute choices that might not be as nutritious.

2. **Shop Smart**: When grocery shopping, focus on fresh foods and whole ingredients. Avoid those with added sugars and high sodium.

3. **Cook at Home**: Preparing meals at home gives you control over ingredients and helps you better manage what you consume.

4. **Listen to Your Body**: Pay attention to how different foods make you feel. This can guide you in adjusting your diet to better suit your health needs.

Balancing your meals is both a science and an art. It requires a thoughtful approach to what you eat and when you eat it. By incorporating a variety of food groups and being mindful of portions and timing, you can transform your meals from mere eating to nourishing your body and enriching your life. Each balanced meal is a step toward better health and enhanced well-being, ensuring that you're not only satisfied but also nourished from the inside out.

3. Setting Up for Success

Embarking on a journey of healthier eating and a balanced lifestyle isn't just about choosing the right foods; it's also about creating an environment that supports these choices. Setting up for success is akin to planting a garden. Just as a gardener cultivates the soil, sows the seeds, and ensures the right conditions for growth, you too must prepare your kitchen and your routines to nurture your nutritional goals. This chapter is dedicated to laying the groundwork for a lifestyle that fosters healthy eating habits effortlessly.

Think of your kitchen as the heart of your home, where good health begins. It's not only the place where meals are cooked; it's where your intentions for a healthier you take physical shape. By organizing it with care, stocking it with the right tools and ingredients, you turn it into a sanctuary of wellness. Whether it's rearranging your pantry to make healthier options more accessible, choosing the right cooking tools that make meal prep simpler and enjoyable, or understanding how to keep fruits and vegetables fresh longer, each action you take makes your health goals more attainable.

Shopping smart is another cornerstone of dietary success. It's about more than just resisting the allure of unhealthy foods; it's about becoming savvy in selecting ingredients that enrich your body. This means understanding labels, knowing what to buy organic, and when non-organic is just as good. It involves learning how to navigate the supermarket to find the healthiest options, and how to make economically wise choices that are good for both your body and your budget.

Beyond the kitchen and the grocery store, this chapter also explores how to weave time-saving cooking techniques into your busy schedule, ensuring that even on your busiest days, a healthy meal is never out of reach. Each step in this chapter is designed to make healthy eating a natural and enjoyable part of your day. It's about setting up a foundation that will carry your healthy habits forward, making each choice not just easier, but almost instinctive.

Preparing Your Kitchen

Imagine stepping into your kitchen, a space not just for cooking but a haven that supports your journey to better health. Preparing your kitchen is a crucial first step in aligning your environment with your health goals. Like setting the stage for a play, the setup of your kitchen can dramatically influence your daily eating habits, making healthy choices effortless and intuitive.

The Philosophy of a Healthy Kitchen

The concept here is simple: make it easier to eat healthily than not. This involves more than just buying the right foods; it involves setting up your physical space to encourage healthy eating patterns. Every aspect of your kitchen, from the layout of your pantry to the tools on your counter, can contribute to your wellness journey.

Optimizing Your Space

Start with decluttering. A cluttered kitchen can lead to a cluttered mind and often, unhealthy food choices. Clear your counters to make room for preparing meals. Keep only the essential tools out in the open. This might include a blender for smoothies, a cutting board for fresh produce, or a slow cooker for preparing nutritious meals with minimal effort.

Strategic Pantry Setup

Organizing your pantry is about making the healthiest choice the easiest choice. Place nutritious snacks at eye level, like nuts, seeds, and dried fruits. Store less healthy treats out of immediate sight to avoid temptation. Stock your shelves with whole grains, legumes, and a variety of herbs and spices that can transform any dish from mundane to mouth-watering without adding excess calories or sodium.

Refrigerator Real Estate

In the fridge, arrange foods so that fruits and vegetables are the first things you see. This not only reminds you to consume your daily dose of vitamins and fibers but also helps reduce food waste. Use clear storage containers to make healthy options immediately visible and accessible. Plan a section for ready-to-eat, pre-cut vegetables, and fruits, making it convenient to choose these over less healthy snacks.

Freezer Management

Your freezer should be your ally in healthy eating, especially when fresh produce is out of season. Freeze fruits for smoothies or to add to yogurt. Keep portions of lean proteins like chicken or fish on hand for quick, healthy meals. Frozen vegetables can be just as nutritious as their fresh counterparts and are great to have available for quick stir-fries or to add substance to soups.

Essential Kitchen Tools

Investing in quality kitchen tools can make meal preparation more enjoyable and less time-consuming. A good set of knives makes chopping vegetables less of a chore. Non-stick cookware can reduce the amount of oil needed for cooking. A pressure cooker or a slow cooker can be excellent for preparing meals in advance, ensuring you always have healthy options on hand even on your busiest days.

Setting Up for Meal Prep

Meal prep is a strategy that pays dividends in your health bank account. Dedicate a part of your kitchen for meal preparation tasks. This could be a corner of your countertop with all necessary tools within reach—cutting boards, mixing bowls, measuring cups, and storage containers. Having this setup invites regular meal prep sessions, which can be essential for a busy week ahead.

The Role of Lighting and Ambiance

The lighting in your kitchen should be bright enough to cook safely and comfortably but also warm and inviting to make the kitchen a pleasant place to be. The more welcoming your kitchen, the more likely you are to spend time there preparing healthy meals. Consider adding some plants or art to make the space more personal and inspiring.

Continuous Improvement

As your dietary needs and cooking skills evolve, so should your kitchen. Periodically reassess your kitchen setup to ensure it continues to meet your needs. Maybe a new dietary preference will necessitate a different set of tools, or perhaps a new cooking technique you've mastered requires rearranging your workspace. Allow your kitchen to grow and adapt with you on your health journey.

By transforming your kitchen into a space that promotes healthy eating, you set yourself up for success. It becomes a place where good choices are easier to make, where healthy eating habits are formed naturally, and where your dietary goals become a practical, visible part of your daily life. Just as a well-tended garden yields a bountiful harvest, a well-prepared kitchen fosters a nourishing and fulfilling dietary lifestyle.

SHOPPING SMART: A GUIDE TO INGREDIENTS

Navigating the supermarket aisles can be akin to exploring a vast treasure map; every choice you make has the potential to contribute positively to your health. Smart shopping is an art form that, when mastered, can transform your pantry into a bastion of nutritional wealth. This sub-chapter aims to arm you with the knowledge and strategies to make every grocery trip an effective and efficient expedition into the world of healthy eating.

Understanding Food Labels

The journey to smart shopping begins with becoming fluent in the language of food labels. Labels are your primary tool for discerning the nutritional value of food. Learn to quickly scan an item for key information: serving size, calories, fats, sodium, sugars, and key nutrients like fiber and protein. Beware of marketing gimmicks that label foods as "natural" or "contains whole grains," which might not always tell the whole nutritional story. Instead, focus on the ingredients list and nutrition facts.

Prioritizing Fresh Ingredients

Whenever possible, steer your cart towards the perimeter of the store. This is typically where the freshest foods—fruits, vegetables, meats, and dairy—are located. Fresh foods are generally less likely to contain the added salts, sugars, and fats found in the more processed foods shelved in the inner aisles. Incorporating a variety of fresh vegetables and fruits into your diet not only enhances flavor but also ensures a broad intake of essential vitamins and minerals.

Choosing Whole Grains

Whole grains should replace refined grains in your diet whenever possible. Whole grains like quinoa, brown rice, whole wheat, and barley retain all parts of the grain, providing more fiber, protein, and nutrients than their refined counterparts. When shopping for bread, cereals, and pasta, always look for the word "whole" in the ingredients list—not just on the front packaging.

Selecting Proteins

Protein is crucial, but the source and quality of protein are equally important. Include a mix of lean animal proteins such as poultry, fish, and eggs, and plant-based proteins such as beans, nuts, and tofu. These sources provide essential amino acids without the high saturated fat content often found in processed meats.

Incorporating Healthy Fats

Not all fats are created equal. Focus on fats that promote health, like those found in avocados, nuts, seeds, and olive oil. These fats can help improve cholesterol levels and offer anti-inflammatory properties. Be wary of products containing trans fats, which can increase heart disease risk. A simple rule of thumb is to avoid or limit anything with "hydrogenated" or "partially hydrogenated" oils in the ingredients list.

Managing Dairy and Dairy Alternatives

If dairy is part of your diet, choose low-fat or fat-free options where possible. These provide the same essential nutrients without the added saturated fat. For those who prefer non-dairy alternatives, ensure they are fortified with calcium and vitamin D, and watch for added sugars—common in flavored varieties.

Being Smart About Snacks

Snacks are often where diets can go astray with high-calorie, low-nutrient options. Look for snacks that contribute to your nutrient intake rather than just filling a craving. Options like yogurt, nuts, fruits, or whole-grain crackers are preferable to chips, candies, or other processed foods.

Decoding Organic and Non-Organic

Organic food is another area to navigate wisely. While organic can mean fewer pesticides and chemicals, it doesn't always mean a product is healthier in terms of calories or fat. Prioritize organic purchases based on foods you consume most often and for products where the organic version may significantly reduce exposure to pesticides, like thin-skinned fruits and vegetables.

Shopping Seasonally and Locally

Purchasing produce that is in season and local is not only more sustainable but often provides better nutrition at a lower cost. Seasonal fruits and vegetables are picked at their peak and don't require long distances for transport, which can degrade nutrients.

Efficient Shopping Practices

Finally, shop with a list and avoid grocery shopping when hungry—a time when high-calorie foods are more tempting. A list helps you stick to your nutritional goals and saves time and money by focusing your purchases on what you really need.

By applying these strategies, your shopping trips can become more than just a routine errand; they become an integral part of your journey towards health. Every item you place in your cart is a choice in favor of your well-being, an investment in your body's health, and a step towards a more vibrant life.

TIME-SAVING COOKING TECHNIQUES

In the rhythm of modern life, time is often at a premium. Cooking, while a fulfilling and essential task, can sometimes feel daunting due to the time it requires. However, with a few strategic techniques, you can transform your kitchen experience, making meal preparation not only quick but also a joy, allowing more time for you to enjoy the fruits of your labor with family and friends.

Batch Cooking: A Weekend Affair

One of the most efficient ways to manage your meals throughout the week is to embrace batch cooking. This involves dedicating a few hours over the weekend to cook large quantities of various staples or complete dishes that store well. Grains like quinoa or brown rice, proteins like roasted chicken, and legumes can be cooked in large amounts and used as bases for multiple meals throughout the week.

Efficient Use of Appliances

Slow Cookers and Pressure Cookers

Slow cookers and pressure cookers are invaluable tools for the time-strapped chef. A slow cooker offers the convenience of "set it and forget it," cooking dishes like stews, soups, and casseroles without needing you to be present. On the flip side, pressure cookers provide the speed to cook meals in a fraction of the time it would normally take. Both methods allow for one-pot meals, significantly reducing both your active cooking and cleaning time.

Blenders and Food Processors

For quick sauces, smoothies, or soup bases, high-powered blenders and food processors can significantly cut down preparation time. These tools excel at reducing vegetables and fruits to purees and sauces, which can be used immediately or stored for future meals.

Advanced Prep Techniques

Pre-Cutting Vegetables

Invest time after shopping to wash and cut vegetables. Store them in clear containers in the fridge, making them easy to grab and use throughout the week. This not only saves time but also increases the likelihood of you reaching for healthy snacks or quickly throwing together a nutritious meal.

Marinating Proteins Before Freezing

Instead of freezing plain proteins, try marinating them first. This not only infuses the proteins with flavor but also means they're ready to cook straight from the thaw. It's a simple step that can add a significant flavor boost to quick meals.

One-Pan and Sheet-Pan Meals

One-pan meals are a revelation for quick and healthy cooking. By combining proteins and vegetables on a single sheet pan and roasting them together in the oven, you can create flavorful, balanced meals with minimal cleanup required. This method also allows the ingredients to enhance each other's flavors as they cook together.

Quick-Cooking Ingredients

Utilizing Quick-Cooking Proteins

Proteins like fish, seafood, or thinly sliced chicken breast can cook in just minutes, much quicker than their thicker or larger counterparts. Incorporating these into your meals can reduce cooking times drastically.

Using Pre-Cooked Ingredients

While fresh is always best, having pre-cooked ingredients on hand can be a lifesaver for last-minute meals. Items like pre-cooked grains or canned beans are great staples that can be quickly transformed into a meal.

Embracing Simplicity

Not every meal needs to be a complex affair. Simple, wholesome ingredients can make satisfying meals with minimal effort. A ripe avocado spread on whole-grain toast, topped with a poached egg and a sprinkle of salt and pepper, is a quick, nutritious meal that is easy to prepare.

Learning and Applying New Skills

Improving your cooking skills can also lead to more efficient cooking. Techniques like proper knife skills can significantly cut down on prep time. Additionally, learning how to sequence your cooking steps — starting with the ingredients that take the longest to cook — can streamline your cooking process.

Make Cooking a Family Affair

Involving family members in the cooking process not only distributes the workload but also makes cooking a more enjoyable and bonding experience. Assign simple tasks like stirring, setting the table, or assembling ingredients to different family members.

By integrating these time-saving techniques into your cooking routine, you make the process less daunting and more enjoyable. These strategies not only help manage time better but also enhance your ability to maintain a healthy diet amidst a busy schedule. The kitchen becomes not just a place of nourishment but a realm of efficiency and creativity.

4. Breakfasts to Kickstart Your Day

Imagine greeting each morning not just with a cup of coffee, but with a meal that truly awakens your body, nourishing it and setting the tone for the day ahead. Breakfast, often cited as the most important meal of the day, holds the key to jumpstarting your metabolism, balancing your energy, and infusing your morning with vitality. This chapter is dedicated to transforming your breakfast from a rushed cup of something on the go to a deliberate, delightful, and nutritious start to your day.

The recipes and ideas you'll discover here are crafted not only to satisfy your taste buds but to align with the principles of the DASH diet—ensuring that each dish is low in sodium and rich in nutrients. We'll explore how a well-composed breakfast can support heart health, manage blood pressure, and provide sustained energy throughout the morning. From smoothies packed with antioxidants to hearty oatmeal or energizing egg dishes, the options are varied and vibrant.

But it's not just about the recipes—it's about understanding how the components of these meals work together to boost your health. You'll learn why incorporating fruits and whole grains can help curb mid-morning cravings and how proteins and healthy fats can keep you feeling fuller longer. This knowledge will empower you to make choices that extend beyond the pages of this book, helping you craft breakfasts that are tailored to your tastes and nutritional needs.

Through this chapter, you'll see how a few thoughtful changes to your morning routine can have profound effects on your well-being. Each recipe is designed to be simple and quick, respecting your time and making it feasible to enjoy a nourishing breakfast even on the busiest mornings. Let's turn the first meal of the day into a cornerstone of daily health and enjoyment, one delightful dish at a time.

AVOCADO TOAST WITH POACHED EGG

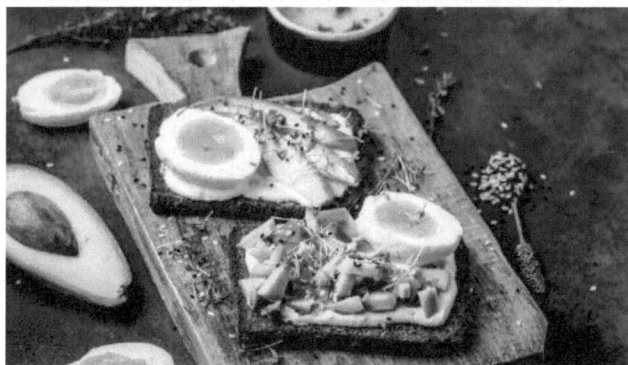

PREPARATION TIME: 10 min **COOKING TIME:** 4 min **MODE OF COOKING:** Toasting/Poaching

INGREDIENTS:

♥1 slice whole-grain bread, toasted;

♥1/2 ripe avocado, mashed;

♥1 egg;

♥1 tsp white vinegar;

♥Salt and pepper to taste;

♥Chili flakes (optional)

DIRECTIONS: 1. Poach egg in simmering water with vinegar for about 4 min; 2. Spread mashed avocado on toasted bread; 3. Top with poached egg; 4. Season with salt, pepper, and chili flakes.

TIPS:

For extra zest, add a squeeze of fresh lime to the avocado.

♥ Garnish with fresh cilantro for an herby touch.

N.V.: Calories: 300, Fat: 20g, Carbs: 23g, Protein: 13g, Sugar: 3g, Sodium: 320 mg, Potassium: 487 mg, Cholesterol: 164 mg, Glucose: 0 mg, Magnesium: 40 mg.

SPINACH AND FETA OMELET

PREPARATION TIME: 10 min **COOKING TIME:** 5 min **MODE OF COOKING:** Sautéing

INGREDIENTS:

♥2 large eggs, beaten;

♥1 cup fresh spinach, chopped;

♥1/4 cup feta cheese, crumbled;

♥1 Tbsp olive oil;

♥Salt and pepper to taste

DIRECTIONS: 1. Heat olive oil in a skillet over medium heat; **2.** Add spinach and sauté until wilted; **3.** Pour eggs over spinach, sprinkle with feta, salt, and pepper; **4.** Cook until eggs are set, fold omelet in half, and serve hot.

TIPS:1. For a creamier texture, whisk a tablespoon of milk into the eggs before cooking. **2.**Serve with a slice of whole-grain toast for a balanced meal.

N.V.: Calories: 250, Fat: 20g, Carbs: 3g, Protein: 13g, Sugar: 1g, Sodium: 410 mg, Potassium: 200 mg, Cholesterol: 370 mg, Glucose: 0 mg, Magnesium: 30 mg.

BANANA ALMOND SMOOTHIE

PREPARATION TIME: 5 min **COOKING TIME:** 0 min **MODE OF COOKING:** Blending

INGREDIENTS:

♥1 ripe banana;

♥1 cup almond milk;

♥1 Tbsp almond butter;

♥1/2 tsp vanilla extract;

♥Ice cubes

DIRECTIONS: 1. Combine all ingredients in a blender; **2.** Blend on high until smooth; **3.** Serve chilled.

TIPS: 1. Add a pinch of cinnamon for extra flavor and health benefits.**2.** Use frozen banana to make the smoothie creamier and colder

N.V.: Calories: 210, Fat: 8g, Carbs: 30g, Protein: 5g, Sugar: 15g, Sodium: 90 mg, Potassium: 422 mg, Cholesterol: 0 mg, Glucose: 0 mg, Magnesium: 50 mg.

BLUEBERRY OATMEAL

PREPARATION TIME: 5 min **COOKING TIME:** 10 min **MODE OF COOKING:** Simmering

INGREDIENTS:

- ♥1/2 cup rolled oats;
- ♥1 cup water;
- ♥1/2 cup fresh blueberries;
- ♥1 Tbsp honey;
- ♥1/4 tsp cinnamon

DIRECTIONS: 1. Bring water to a boil in a small pot; **2.** Add oats and simmer until soft, about 5 min; **3.** Stir in blueberries, honey, and cinnamon; **4.** Cook for another **5** min, then serve.

TIPS:1. Top with a dollop of Greek yogurt for added protein and creaminess.**2.** Sprinkle with chopped nuts for added crunch and nutrients.

N.V.: Calories: 180, Fat: 2g, Carbs: 37g, Protein: 4g, Sugar: 12g, Sodium: 10 mg, Potassium: 90 mg, Cholesterol: 0 mg, Glucose: 0 mg, Magnesium: 60 mg.

CHIA SEED PUDDING

PREPARATION TIME: 10 min **COOKING TIME:** 0 min **MODE OF COOKING:** Refrigerating

INGREDIENTS:

- ♥1/4 cup chia seeds;
- ♥1 cup coconut milk;
- ♥1 Tbsp maple syrup;
- ♥1/2 tsp vanilla extract

DIRECTIONS: 1. Mix all ingredients in a bowl; 2. Stir well to combine; 3. Refrigerate overnight; 4. Serve chilled with optional toppings like nuts or fruit.

TIPS: 1. For a tropical twist, replace maple syrup with honey and add a layer of mango puree before refrigerating. **2.** Stir in a spoonful of cocoa powder for a chocolate version.

N.V.: Calories: 280, Fat: 18g, Carbs: 25g, Protein: 5g, Sugar: 12g, Sodium: 15 mg, Potassium: 240 mg, Cholesterol: 0 mg, Glucose: 0 mg, Magnesium: 70 mg.

SWEET POTATO HASH WITH EGGS

PREPARATION TIME: 15 min **COOKING TIME:** 20 min **MODE OF COOKING:** Sautéing

INGREDIENTS:

- ♥2 medium sweet potatoes, diced;
- ♥1 red bell pepper, chopped;
- ♥1 onion, chopped;
- ♥2 cloves garlic, minced;
- ♥4 eggs;
- ♥2 Tbsp olive oil;
- ♥Salt and pepper to taste;
- ♥1/2 tsp smoked paprika

DIRECTIONS: 1. Heat olive oil in a large skillet over medium heat; **2.** Add sweet potatoes, bell pepper, onion, and garlic; sauté until potatoes are tender, about 15 min; **3.** Make four wells in the hash, crack an egg into each well; **4.** Cover and cook until eggs are set, about 5 min; **5.** Season with salt, pepper, and smoked paprika before serving.

TIPS: 1. Add a splash of hot sauce for a spicy kick. **2.** Garnish with fresh parsley or cilantro for added freshness.

N.V.: Calories: 320, Fat: 18g, Carbs: 27g, Protein: 12g, Sugar: 7g, Sodium: 150 mg, Potassium: 762 mg, Cholesterol: 210 mg, Glucose: 0 mg, Magnesium: 45 mg.

GREEK YOGURT PARFAIT

PREPARATION TIME: 5 min **COOKING TIME:** 0 min **MODE OF COOKING:** Assembling

INGREDIENTS:

- ♥1 cup Greek yogurt;
- ♥1/4 cup granola;
- ♥1/2 cup mixed berries (strawberries, blueberries, raspberries);
- ♥1 Tbsp honey

DIRECTIONS: 1. Layer half of the Greek yogurt in a glass; **2.** Add half of the granola and half of the berries; **3.** Repeat the layering with the remaining yogurt, granola, and berries; **4.** Drizzle honey on top before serving.

TIPS: 1. For a crunchier texture, toast the granola in a dry pan until golden. **2.** Swap honey with agave syrup for a vegan alternative.

N.V.: Calories: 290, Fat: 4g, Carbs: 46g, Protein: 20g, Sugar: 32g, Sodium: 70 mg, Potassium: 345 mg, Cholesterol: 10 mg, Glucose: 0 mg, Magnesium: 18 mg.

COTTAGE CHEESE AND PINEAPPLE BREAKFAST BOWLS

PREPARATION TIME: 5 min **COOKING TIME:** 0 min **MODE OF COOKING:** Mixing

INGREDIENTS:

- ♥1 cup low-fat cottage cheese;
- ♥1/2 cup chopped pineapple;
- ♥1/4 cup chopped walnuts;
- ♥1 tsp chia seeds;
- ♥1 Tbsp honey

DIRECTIONS: 1. Place cottage cheese in a serving bowl; **2.** Top with pineapple, walnuts, and chia seeds; **3.** Drizzle with honey before serving.

TIPS: 1. Mix in a teaspoon of vanilla extract to the cottage cheese for extra flavor.**2.** Replace pineapple with mango for a different tropical twist.

N.V.: Calories: 350, Fat: 15g, Carbs: 35g, Protein: 20g, Sugar: 25g, Sodium: 500 mg, Potassium: 200 mg, Cholesterol: 5 mg, Glucose: 0 mg, Magnesium: 30 mg.

TURKEY AND SPINACH SCRAMBLED EGGS

PREPARATION TIME: 5 min **COOKING TIME:** 10 min **MODE OF COOKING:** Scrambling

INGREDIENTS:

- ♥4 eggs;
- ♥1/4 lb cooked turkey breast, chopped;
- ♥1 cup fresh spinach, chopped;
- ♥1 Tbsp olive oil;
- ♥Salt and pepper to taste

DIRECTIONS: 1. Heat olive oil in a skillet over medium heat; **2.** Add turkey and spinach and cook until spinach is wilted; **3.** Beat eggs and pour over turkey mixture; **4.** Cook, stirring frequently, until eggs are scrambled and cooked through; 5. Season with salt and pepper.

TIPS: 1. Enhance flavor with a sprinkle of grated Parmesan. **2.** Serve with a side of avocado slices for healthy fats.

N.V.: Calories: 230, Fat: 14g, Carbs: 2g, Protein: 24g, Sugar: 1g, Sodium: 190 mg, Potassium: 290 mg, Cholesterol: 372 mg, Glucose: 0 mg, Magnesium: 50 mg.

QUINOA AND BERRY BREAKFAST BOWL

PREPARATION TIME: 5 min **COOKING TIME:** 15 min **MODE OF COOKING:** Boiling

INGREDIENTS:

- ♥1/2 cup quinoa;
- ♥1 cup water;
- ♥1/2 cup mixed berries;
- ♥1 Tbsp sliced almonds;
- ♥1 Tbsp maple syrup

DIRECTIONS: 1. Rinse quinoa under cold water; **2.** Bring water to a boil in a small pot, add quinoa, reduce heat, and simmer covered until water is absorbed, about 15 min; **3.** Fluff quinoa with a fork and mix in berries and almonds; **4.** Drizzle with maple syrup before serving.

TIPS: 1. Toast the almonds before adding them to the bowl for extra crunch.**2.** Drizzle with a little bit of almond milk for added moisture and flavor.

N.V.: Calories: 295, Fat: 5g, Carbs: 54g, Protein: 8g, Sugar: 15g, Sodium: 13 mg, Potassium: 222 mg, Cholesterol: 0 mg, Glucose: 0 mg, Magnesium: 78 mg.

TOFU AND VEGETABLE STIR-FRY

PREPARATION TIME: 10 min **COOKING TIME:** 10 min **MODE OF COOKING:** Stir-frying

INGREDIENTS:

- ♥1/2 lb firm tofu, cubed;
- ♥1 cup mixed bell peppers, sliced;
- ♥1/2 cup broccoli florets;
- ♥2 Tbsp soy sauce;
- ♥1 Tbsp sesame oil;
- ♥1 clove garlic, minced

DIRECTIONS: 1. Heat sesame oil in a large skillet over medium-high heat; **2.** Add garlic, tofu, and vegetables; stir-fry until vegetables are tender and tofu is golden, about 10 min; **3.** Stir in soy sauce and cook for another minute.

TIPS: 1. Add a splash of chili sauce for a spicy version.**2.** Garnish with toasted sesame seeds for a nutty finish.

N.V.: Calories: 200, Fat: 12g, Carbs: 10g, Protein: 12g, Sugar: 4g, Sodium: 660 mg, Potassium: 300 mg, Cholesterol: 0 mg, Glucose: 0 mg, Magnesium: 35 mg.

APPLE CINNAMON QUINOA BOWL

PREPARATION TIME: 5 min **COOKING TIME:** 20 min **MODE OF COOKING:** Boiling

INGREDIENTS:

- ♥1/2 cup quinoa;
- ♥1 cup water;
- ♥1 apple, diced;
- ♥1/2 tsp cinnamon;
- ♥1 Tbsp almond butter;
- ♥1 tsp honey

DIRECTIONS: 1. Rinse quinoa under cold running water; **2.** Combine quinoa, water, and cinnamon in a saucepan and bring to a boil; **3.** Reduce heat to low, cover, and simmer until quinoa is cooked, about 15 min; **4.** Stir in apple, almond butter, and honey; 5. Serve warm.

TIPS: 1. For extra protein, stir in a scoop of vanilla protein powder.**2.** Serve topped with a sprinkle of flax seeds for additional Omega-3s.

N.V.: Calories: 315, Fat: 8g, Carbs: 55g, Protein: 8g, Sugar: 12g, Sodium: 7 mg, Potassium: 239 mg, Cholesterol: 0 mg, Glucose: 0 mg, Magnesium: 118 mg.

PEANUT BUTTER BANANA OAT SMOOTHIE

PREPARATION TIME: 5 min **COOKING TIME:** 0 min **MODE OF COOKING:** Blending

INGREDIENTS:

- ♥1 banana;
- ♥1/4 cup oats;
- ♥1 Tbsp peanut butter;
- ♥1 cup almond milk;
- ♥1/2 tsp vanilla extract

DIRECTIONS: 1. Place all ingredients in a blender; **2.** Blend on high until smooth and creamy; **3.** Serve immediately.

TIPS: 1. Add a dash of cinnamon for a warming flavor.**2.**Use frozen banana to enhance the smoothie's creaminess without needing ice.

N.V.: Calories: 280, Fat: 9g, Carbs: 45g, Protein: 8g, Sugar: 15g, Sodium: 150 mg, Potassium: 422 mg, Cholesterol: 0 mg, Glucose: 0 mg, Magnesium: 72 mg.

MEDITERRANEAN VEGETABLE FRITTATA

PREPARATION TIME: 10 min **COOKING TIME:** 20 min **MODE OF COOKING:** Baking

INGREDIENTS:

- ♥4 eggs;
- ♥1/2 cup diced tomatoes;
- ♥1/4 cup chopped spinach;
- ♥1/4 cup crumbled feta cheese;
- ♥1/4 cup diced onions;
- ♥1 Tbsp olive oil;
- ♥Salt and pepper to taste

DIRECTIONS: 1. Preheat oven to 375°F (190°C); **2.** Sauté onions and spinach in olive oil until soft; **3.** Beat eggs and mix with tomatoes, cooked onions, and spinach; **4.** Pour into a greased baking dish, sprinkle with feta; 5. Bake for 20 min or until set.

TIPS: 1. Serve with a side of mixed greens dressed with olive oil and lemon for a refreshing contrast. **2.** Add sliced olives or capers for an extra Mediterranean touch.

N.V.: Calories: 220, Fat: 15g, Carbs: 8g, Protein: 14g, Sugar: 4g, Sodium: 310 mg, Potassium: 240 mg, Cholesterol: 370 mg, Glucose: 0 mg, Magnesium: 28 mg.

RASPBERRY CHIA OVERNIGHT OATS

PREPARATION TIME: 5 min **COOKING TIME:** 0 min **MODE OF COOKING:** Refrigerating

INGREDIENTS:

- ♥1/2 cup rolled oats;
- ♥1 Tbsp chia seeds;
- ♥1/2 cup raspberries;
- ♥3/4 cup almond milk;
- ♥1 tsp honey

DIRECTIONS: 1. Combine all ingredients in a mason jar; **2.** Stir until well mixed; **3.** Seal and refrigerate overnight; **4.** Serve cold, stirred.

TIPS: 1. Top with a handful of toasted coconut flakes for texture and tropical flavor.**2** Mix in a spoonful of cocoa powder for a chocolatey twist.

N.V.: Calories: 255, Fat: 7g, Carbs: 39g, Protein: 8g, Sugar: 9g, Sodium: 95 mg, Potassium: 200 mg, Cholesterol: 0 mg, Glucose: 0 mg, Magnesium: 95 mg.

SPICED PUMPKIN PANCAKES

PREPARATION TIME: 10 min **COOKING TIME:** 10 min **MODE OF COOKING:** Griddling

INGREDIENTS:

- ♥1 cup all-purpose flour;
- ♥1/2 cup pumpkin puree;
- ♥1 cup milk;
- ♥1 egg;
- ♥2 Tbsp maple syrup;
- ♥1 tsp baking powder;
- ♥1/2 tsp cinnamon;
- ♥1/4 tsp nutmeg;
- ♥Butter for cooking

DIRECTIONS: 1. Combine flour, baking powder, cinnamon, and nutmeg in a mixing bowl; **2.** In another bowl, mix milk, pumpkin puree, egg, and maple syrup; **3.** Gradually add the wet ingredients to the dry, mixing until just combined; **4.** Heat a griddle over medium heat and grease with butter; **5.** Pour 1/4 cup batter for each pancake, cook until bubbles form on the surface, then flip and cook until golden.

TIPS: 1. Serve with a dollop of whipped cream and a sprinkle of cinnamon sugar for a festive touch. **2.** Pair with a cup of hot apple cider for a cozy breakfast experience.

N.V.: Calories: 260, Fat: 5g, Carbs: 45g, Protein: 8g, Sugar: 12g, Sodium: 220 mg, Potassium: 199 mg, Cholesterol: 55 mg, Glucose: 0 mg, Magnesium: 30 mg.

5. LUNCHES FOR BUSY BEES

In the rhythm of our bustling daily lives, lunch often becomes an overlooked meal, hastily assembled from leftovers, grabbed on the go, or, worse yet, skipped altogether. But let's reimagine this midday pause not just as a necessity but as a delightful interlude—a moment to refuel both body and spirit amid our hectic schedules.

Imagine sitting down to a meal that feels like a breath of fresh air, a nutritious spread that comes together quickly yet satisfies your taste buds and powers you through the rest of your day. Whether you're a corporate warrior tethered to your desk, a busy parent juggling the endless demands of home and work, or a creative soul constantly on the move, the recipes in this chapter are designed with your lifestyle in mind.

These dishes strike a harmonious balance between convenience and health, without requiring long hours in the kitchen. They are crafted to be prepared ahead, easily portable, and adaptable to the vibrant, ever-changing tapestry of daily life. Each recipe is a building block towards maintaining a balanced diet, even when time is a precious commodity.

Consider the joy of unveiling a Mason jar layered with vibrant greens, protein-packed grains, and a zesty dressing that enlivens the senses and shakes off the midday slump. Or imagine the comfort of a warm, homemade soup that tastes like it simmered for hours but actually came together in a flash one leisurely Sunday afternoon, ready to be reheated and enjoyed any day of the week.

Lunch should be a meal that you look forward to—a moment that is as nourishing for the mind as it is for the body. It's a chance to slow down, even if just for a little while, to savor flavors that are both comforting and invigorating, and to remind ourselves that eating well is a form of self-respect and love.

So, let's set aside the notion that lunches are too cumbersome to enjoy amid busy schedules. With a little planning and a dash of creativity, you can transform this overlooked meal into a highlight of your day, a true feast for the senses that energizes, satisfies, and, most importantly, brings a moment of well-deserved pleasure to your busy day.

Spicy Tuna Quinoa Salad

PREPARATION TIME: 15 min **COOKING TIME:** 0 min **MODE OF COOKING:** Mixing

INGREDIENTS:

- ♥1 can tuna in water, drained;
- ♥1 cup cooked quinoa;
- ♥1/2 cucumber, diced;

- ♥1/2 red bell pepper, diced;
- ♥1/4 red onion, finely chopped;
- ♥2 Tbsp mayonnaise;
- ♥1 tsp sriracha sauce;
- ♥1 Tbsp lemon juice;
- ♥Salt and pepper to taste

DIRECTIONS: 1. In a large bowl, combine tuna, quinoa, cucumber, bell pepper, and onion; 2. In a small bowl, mix mayonnaise, sriracha, and lemon juice; 3. Pour dressing over tuna mixture and toss to combine; 4. Season with salt and pepper.

TIPS: 1 Adjust the amount of sriracha based on spice preference. **2** Serve over a bed of fresh spinach for extra greens.

N.V.: Calories: 310, Fat: 9g, Carbs: 33g, Protein: 23g, Sugar: 4g, Sodium: 460 mg, Potassium: 520 mg, Cholesterol: 30 mg, Glucose: 0 mg, Magnesium: 80 mg.

Grilled Chicken Caesar Wrap

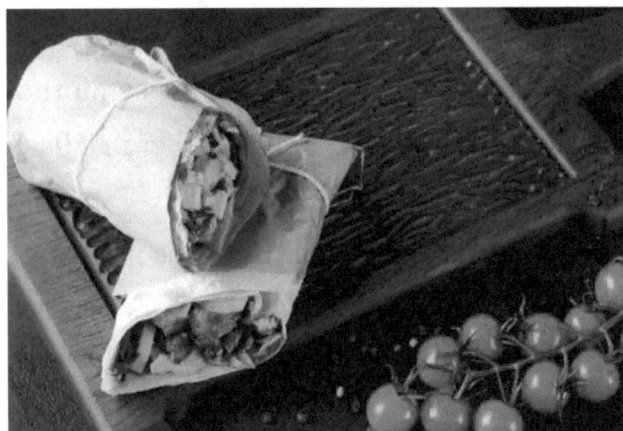

PREPARATION TIME: 10 min **COOKING TIME:** 10 min **MODE OF COOKING:** Grilling

INGREDIENTS:
- ♥2 chicken breasts;
- ♥2 large whole wheat wraps;
- ♥1/2 cup Caesar dressing;
- ♥1 cup romaine lettuce, chopped;
- ♥1/4 cup Parmesan cheese, shaved;
- ♥1 tsp olive oil;
- ♥Salt and pepper to taste

DIRECTIONS: 1. Season chicken breasts with salt and pepper; 2. Grill chicken over medium heat until cooked through, about 5 min per side; 3. Slice chicken and place on wraps; 4. Top with lettuce, Parmesan, and Caesar dressing; 5. Roll wraps tightly and cut in half.

TIPS: 1 Use low-fat Caesar dressing to reduce calories. **2** Add sliced avocado for extra creaminess and nutrients.

N.V.: Calories: 450, Fat: 22g, Carbs: 33g, Protein: 32g, Sugar: 3g, Sodium: 790 mg, Potassium: 450 mg, Cholesterol: 80 mg, Glucose: 0 mg, Magnesium: 50 mg.

Avocado & Chickpea Hummus Wrap

PREPARATION TIME: 10 min **COOKING TIME:** 0 min **MODE OF COOKING:** Assembling

INGREDIENTS:

- ♥2 whole wheat wraps;
- ♥1 ripe avocado, mashed;
- ♥1 cup canned chickpeas, rinsed and mashed;
- ♥1/2 carrot, grated;
- ♥1/4 cup red cabbage, shredded;
- ♥1 Tbsp olive oil;
- ♥1 tsp lemon juice;
- ♥Salt and pepper to taste

DIRECTIONS: 1. Combine mashed avocado and chickpeas in a bowl; 2. Stir in olive oil, lemon juice, salt, and pepper; 3. Spread the mixture on wraps; 4. Top with grated carrot and shredded cabbage; 5. Roll tightly and slice in half.

TIPS: 1 Add a sprinkle of chili flakes for a spicy kick. **2** Drizzle with tahini for an extra flavor layer.

N.V.: Calories: 410, Fat: 20g, Carbs: 50g, Protein: 12g, Sugar: 5g, Sodium: 420 mg, Potassium: 690 mg, Cholesterol: 0 mg, Glucose: 0 mg, Magnesium: 60 mg.

Beet and Goat Cheese Arugula Salad

PREPARATION TIME: 10 min **COOKING TIME:** 0 min **MODE OF COOKING:** Mixing

INGREDIENTS:

- ♥3 beets, cooked and sliced;
- ♥2 cups arugula;
- ♥1/2 cup goat cheese, crumbled;
- ♥1/4 cup walnuts, chopped;
- ♥2 Tbsp balsamic vinegar;
- ♥1 Tbsp olive oil;
- ♥Salt and pepper to taste

DIRECTIONS: 1. Place arugula on a serving plate; 2. Top with sliced beets, goat cheese, and walnuts; 3. Whisk together balsamic vinegar, olive oil, salt, and pepper; 4. Drizzle dressing over the salad before serving.

TIPS: 1 Roast beets ahead of time for enhanced sweetness. **2** Substitute walnuts with pecans if preferred.

N.V.: Calories: 290, Fat: 19g, Carbs: 21g, Protein: 9g, Sugar: 14g, Sodium: 270 mg, Potassium: 540 mg, Cholesterol: 13 mg, Glucose: 0 mg, Magnesium: 40 mg.

Lemon Herb Grilled Salmon

PREPARATION TIME: 10 min **COOKING TIME:** 10 min **MODE OF COOKING:** Grilling

INGREDIENTS:

- ♥4 salmon fillets, 4 oz each;
- ♥2 lemons, one juiced and one sliced;
- ♥2 Tbsp olive oil;
- ♥1 Tbsp fresh dill, chopped;
- ♥1 Tbsp fresh parsley, chopped;
- ♥Salt and pepper to taste

DIRECTIONS: 1. Preheat grill to medium-high heat; 2. In a small bowl, mix lemon juice, olive oil, dill, parsley, salt, and pepper; 3. Brush salmon with lemon herb mixture; 4. Grill salmon, skin-side down, until cooked through, about 5 min per side; 5. Serve with lemon slices.

TIPS: 1 Ensure grill is well-oiled to prevent sticking. **2** Perfect with a side of steamed asparagus.

N.V.: Calories: 300, Fat: 18g, Carbs: 2g, Protein: 30g, Sugar: 1g, Sodium: 75 mg, Potassium: 830 mg, Cholesterol: 85 mg, Glucose: 0 mg, Magnesium: 50 mg.

Sweet Potato & Black Bean Burrito

PREPARATION TIME: 15 min **COOKING TIME:** 25 min **MODE OF COOKING:** Roasting, Assembling

INGREDIENTS:

- ♥2 medium sweet potatoes, peeled and cubed;
- ♥1 can black beans, drained and rinsed;
- ♥1/2 cup corn;
- ♥1 tsp cumin;
- ♥1/2 tsp chili powder;
- ♥4 whole wheat tortillas;
- ♥1/2 cup shredded cheddar cheese;
- ♥1 avocado, sliced;
- ♥1 lime, juiced;
- ♥Salt and pepper to taste;
- ♥1 Tbsp olive oil

DIRECTIONS: 1. Preheat oven to 400°F (204°C); 2. Toss sweet potatoes with olive oil, cumin, chili powder, salt, and pepper; 3. Roast for 25 min until tender; 4. Warm tortillas; 5. Divide sweet potatoes, black beans, corn, cheese, and avocado among tortillas; 6. Squeeze lime over filling, roll up burritos.

TIPS: 1 Add a dollop of Greek yogurt for creaminess. **2** Wrap burritos in foil for an easy on-the-go lunch.

N.V.: Calories: 450, Fat: 18g, Carbs: 60g, Protein: 14g, Sugar: 5g, Sodium: 390 mg, Potassium: 1012 mg, Cholesterol: 30 mg, Glucose: 0 mg, Magnesium: 85 mg.

Pesto Pasta Salad with Cherry Tomatoes

PREPARATION TIME: 10 min **COOKING TIME:** 10 min **MODE OF COOKING:** Boiling
INGREDIENTS:

♥2 cups whole wheat pasta, cooked and cooled;

♥1/2 cup pesto;

♥1 cup cherry tomatoes, halved;

♥1/4 cup pine nuts, toasted;

♥1/4 cup Parmesan cheese, grated;

♥Salt and pepper to taste

DIRECTIONS: 1. In a large bowl, combine pasta, pesto, cherry tomatoes, and pine nuts; 2. Toss until well coated; 3. Season with salt and pepper; 4. Sprinkle with Parmesan cheese before serving.

TIPS: 1 Chill the salad before serving for enhanced flavors. **2** Substitute arugula for basil in pesto for a peppery twist.

N.V.: Calories: 380, Fat: 22g, Carbs: 35g, Protein: 10g, Sugar: 3g, Sodium: 330 mg, Potassium: 255 mg, Cholesterol: 4 mg, Glucose: 0 mg, Magnesium: 45 mg.

Asian Chicken Salad with Ginger Sesame Dressing

PREPARATION TIME: 20 min **COOKING TIME:** 0 min **MODE OF COOKING:** Mixing

INGREDIENTS:

- ♥2 cups cooked chicken, shredded;
- ♥2 cups mixed greens;
- ♥1/2 cup shredded carrots;
- ♥1/4 cup slivered almonds;
- ♥2 Tbsp sesame seeds;
- ♥1/4 cup soy sauce;
- ♥1 Tbsp sesame oil;
- ♥1 Tbsp honey;
- ♥1 tsp fresh ginger, grated;
- ♥1 garlic clove, minced

DIRECTIONS: 1. In a large bowl, combine chicken, mixed greens, carrots, almonds, and sesame seeds; 2. In a small bowl, whisk together soy sauce, sesame oil, honey, ginger, and garlic; 3. Drizzle dressing over salad and toss to coat.

TIPS: 1 Garnish with mandarin orange segments for extra zest. **2** Serve chilled for a refreshing lunch option.

N.V.: Calories: 310, Fat: 15g, Carbs: 15g, Protein: 27g, Sugar: 7g, Sodium: 790 mg, Potassium: 440 mg, Cholesterol: 60 mg, Glucose: 0 mg, Magnesium: 60 mg.

Roasted Beet and Goat Cheese Sandwich

PREPARATION TIME: 15 min **COOKING TIME:** 30 min **MODE OF COOKING:** Roasting, Assembling

INGREDIENTS:

- ♥2 medium beets, roasted and sliced;
- ♥4 oz goat cheese;
- ♥2 cups arugula;
- ♥4 slices whole grain bread;
- ♥1 Tbsp olive oil;
- ♥1 Tbsp balsamic glaze

DIRECTIONS: 1. Preheat oven to 375°F (190°C); 2. Wrap beets in foil, roast until tender, about 30 min; 3. Spread goat cheese on bread slices; 4. Layer roasted beets and arugula on two bread slices; 5. Drizzle with olive oil and balsamic glaze; 6. Top with remaining bread slices to form sandwiches.

TIPS: 1 Add walnut pieces for crunch and extra nutrition. **2** Press sandwich in a panini press for a warm, crispy texture.

N.V.: Calories: 420, Fat: 22g, Carbs: 39g, Protein: 17g, Sugar: 10g, Sodium: 460 mg, Potassium: 365 mg, Cholesterol: 30 mg, Glucose: 0 mg, Magnesium: 50 mg.

Smoked Turkey and Cranberry Ciabatta

PREPARATION TIME: 10 min **COOKING TIME:** 0 min **MODE OF COOKING:** Assembling

INGREDIENTS:

- ♥1 ciabatta loaf, cut into 4 sandwiches;
- ♥8 oz smoked turkey, sliced;
- ♥1/4 cup cranberry sauce;
- ♥1/4 cup arugula;
- ♥4 Tbsp cream cheese

DIRECTIONS: 1. Spread cream cheese on each ciabatta slice; 2. Layer with smoked turkey and a spoonful of cranberry sauce; 3. Add arugula; 4. Assemble sandwiches and serve.

TIPS: 1 Toast ciabatta slices lightly for added crunch. **2** Swap arugula with spinach for a milder taste.

N.V.: Calories: 360, Fat: 12g, Carbs: 45g, Protein: 24g, Sugar: 8g, Sodium: 900 mg, Potassium: 300 mg, Cholesterol: 55 mg, Glucose: 0 mg, Magnesium: 40 mg.

Caprese Salad with Balsamic Reduction

PREPARATION TIME: 10 min **COOKING TIME:** 10 min **MODE OF COOKING:** Reducing

INGREDIENTS:

- ♥3 large tomatoes, sliced;
- ♥8 oz mozzarella cheese, sliced;
- ♥1/4 cup fresh basil leaves;
- ♥2 Tbsp balsamic vinegar;
- ♥1 Tbsp honey;
- ♥Salt and pepper to taste;
- ♥1 Tbsp olive oil

DIRECTIONS: 1. Arrange tomato and mozzarella slices on a plate, alternating and overlapping; 2. Scatter basil leaves over the top; 3. In a small saucepan, heat balsamic vinegar and honey, simmer until thickened, about 10 min; 4. Drizzle olive oil and balsamic reduction over salad; 5. Season with salt and pepper.

TIPS: 1 For best flavor, use high-quality, aged balsamic vinegar. **2** Serve as a refreshing starter or light lunch.

N.V.: Calories: 280, Fat: 18g, Carbs: 14g, Protein: 16g, Sugar: 10g, Sodium: 420 mg, Potassium: 340 mg, Cholesterol: 44 mg, Glucose: 0 mg, Magnesium: 30 mg.

Lentil Soup with Spinach and Lemon

PREPARATION TIME: 10 min **COOKING TIME:** 30 min **MODE OF COOKING:** Simmering

INGREDIENTS:

- ♥1 cup dried lentils, rinsed;
- ♥4 cups vegetable broth;
- ♥1 onion, chopped;
- ♥2 carrots, diced;
- ♥2 garlic cloves, minced;
- ♥1 tsp cumin;
- ♥2 cups fresh spinach;
- ♥1 lemon, juiced;
- ♥Salt and pepper to taste;
- ♥1 Tbsp olive oil

DIRECTIONS: 1. In a large pot, heat olive oil over medium heat; 2. Add onions, carrots, and garlic, sauté until softened; 3. Stir in lentils, broth, and cumin; 4. Simmer until lentils are tender, about 30 min; 5. Stir in spinach and lemon juice; 6. Season with salt and pepper; 7. Serve hot.

TIPS: 1 Top with a dollop of yogurt for creaminess. **2** Serve with crusty bread for a hearty meal.

N.V.: Calories: 250, Fat: 4g, Carbs: 38g, Protein: 14g, Sugar: 4g, Sodium: 300 mg, Potassium: 730 mg, Cholesterol: 0 mg, Glucose: 0 mg, Magnesium: 80 mg.

Grilled Vegetable and Hummus Pita

PREPARATION TIME: 15 min **COOKING TIME:** 10 min **MODE OF COOKING:** Grilling, Assembling

INGREDIENTS:

- ♥2 whole wheat pitas;
- ♥1 zucchini, sliced;
- ♥1 yellow squash, sliced;
- ♥1 red bell pepper, sliced;
- ♥1/4 cup hummus;
- ♥1 Tbsp olive oil;
- ♥Salt and pepper to taste

DIRECTIONS: 1. Preheat grill to medium-high; 2. Brush vegetables with olive oil, season with salt and pepper; 3. Grill vegetables until charred and tender, about 5 min per side; 4. Spread hummus inside pitas; 5. Stuff with grilled vegetables; 6. Serve warm.

TIPS: 1 Add feta cheese for extra flavor. **2** Drizzle with tahini for a creamy finish.

N.V.: Calories: 330, Fat: 12g, Carbs: 47g, Protein: 9g, Sugar: 8g, Sodium: 390 mg, Potassium: 510 mg, Cholesterol: 0 mg, Glucose: 0 mg, Magnesium: 72 mg.

Soba Noodle Salad with Edamame and Ginger Dressing

PREPARATION TIME: 10 min **COOKING TIME:** 5 min **MODE OF COOKING:** Boiling

INGREDIENTS:

- ♥1 package soba noodles;
- ♥1 cup shelled edamame;
- ♥1 carrot, julienned;
- ♥1 cucumber, julienned;
- ♥1/4 cup soy sauce;
- ♥1 Tbsp fresh ginger, grated;
- ♥1 Tbsp honey;
- ♥1 Tbsp rice vinegar;
- ♥1 tsp sesame oil

DIRECTIONS: 1. Cook soba noodles according to package instructions, rinse under cold water; 2. In a large bowl, combine noodles, edamame, carrot, and cucumber; 3. In a small bowl, whisk together soy sauce, ginger, honey, vinegar, and sesame oil; 4. Pour dressing over noodle mixture, toss to coat; 5. Chill before serving.

TIPS: 1 Top with sesame seeds for extra crunch. **2** Add shredded chicken for more protein.

N.V.: Calories: 320, Fat: 5g, Carbs: 55g, Protein: 15g, Sugar: 9g, Sodium: 630 mg, Potassium: 400 mg, Cholesterol: 0 mg, Glucose: 0 mg, Magnesium: 75 mg.

6. Dinners: Simple and Satisfying

As the sun dips below the horizon and the day winds down, the evening meal becomes not just a time to nourish our bodies but also an opportunity to reconnect with ourselves and our loved ones. Dinner, in its quintessential form, is more than food on a plate; it's a moment to decompress, to savor and to relish the quiet or the chaos of family life. This chapter is dedicated to transforming dinner into an effortlessly enjoyable part of your day.

The recipes you'll find here are designed with both simplicity and satisfaction in mind. They cater to the seasoned home cook looking for something straightforward yet delicious, as well as to the culinary novice who might be tentative about complex recipes. Each dish is crafted to minimize kitchen time and maximize flavor, using ingredients that bring comfort and a touch of creativity to your table.

Imagine dishes that cook in harmony with your evening routine, whether that means a slow cooker simmering as you help with homework, a one-pan meal that cuts down on washing up so you can spend a little longer unwinding, or a quick and vibrant stir-fry that comes together as quickly as your day changes pace. These meals are about making dinner a feasible, enjoyable endeavor that complements your lifestyle rather than complicates it.

In this chapter, you'll discover that a nourishing, fulfilling dinner doesn't require hours of preparation. It's entirely possible to prepare a meal that satisfies the soul as well as the palate without a sink full of dishes afterward. From hearty soups that hug you from the inside out to grilled meats and vegetables that barely need a watchful eye, the focus is on low-effort, high-reward meals.

Let each recipe guide you through evenings filled with flavor without forfeiting moments of relaxation. After all, the essence of a great dinner lies not only in the taste and health benefits it offers but also in the ease and joy with which it can be prepared. Embrace these recipes as your toolkit for ending each day on a delicious note, knowing that something simple and satisfying is always within reach.

Herb-Crusted Salmon with Asparagus

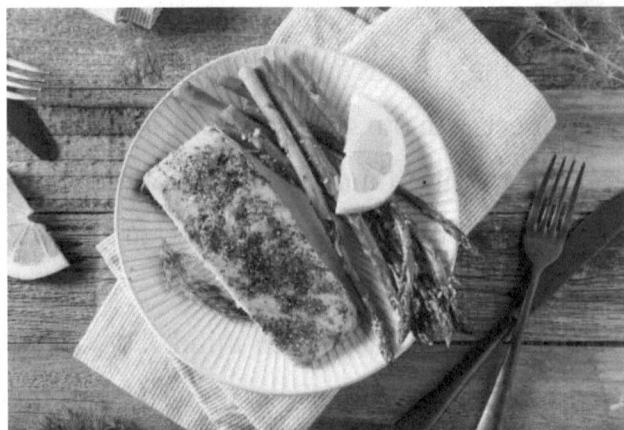

PREPARATION TIME: 10 min **COOKING TIME:** 20 min **MODE OF COOKING:** Baking

INGREDIENTS:

- ♥4 salmon fillets, 6 oz each;
- ♥1 bunch asparagus, trimmed;
- ♥2 Tbsp olive oil;
- ♥1 tsp dried basil;
- ♥1 tsp dried oregano;
- ♥1/2 tsp garlic powder;
- ♥Salt and pepper to taste

DIRECTIONS: 1 Preheat oven to 400°F (204°C); **2** Mix olive oil, basil, oregano, garlic powder, salt, and pepper in a bowl; **3** Brush mixture on salmon and asparagus; **4** Place on a baking sheet and bake for 20 min.

TIPS: 1 Serve with a wedge of lemon for added zest. **2** Pair with quinoa for a complete meal.

N.V.: Calories: 345, Fat: 22g, Carbs: 5g, Protein: 33g, Sugar: 1g, Sodium: 75 mg, Potassium: 834 mg, Cholesterol: 88 mg, Glucose: 0 mg, Magnesium: 50 mg.

Garlic Lemon Chicken with Green Beans

PREPARATION TIME: 10 min **COOKING TIME:** 20 min **MODE OF COOKING:** Roasting

INGREDIENTS:

- ♥4 chicken breasts;
- ♥1 lb green beans, ends trimmed;
- ♥4 garlic cloves, minced;
- ♥2 lemons, one sliced, one juiced;
- ♥3 Tbsp olive oil;
- ♥Salt and pepper to taste

DIRECTIONS: 1 Preheat oven to 400°F (204°C); **2** Place chicken and green beans on a baking sheet; **3** Mix olive oil, lemon juice, garlic, salt, and pepper; **4** Pour mixture over chicken and beans; **5** Top with lemon slices; **6** Roast for 20 min until chicken is cooked.

TIPS: 1 Use parchment paper for easy cleanup. **2** Add capers for a tangy twist.

N.V.: Calories: 290, Fat: 12g, Carbs: 8g, Protein: 35g, Sugar: 2g, Sodium: 85 mg, Potassium: 650 mg, Cholesterol: 85 mg, Glucose: 0 mg, Magnesium: 55 mg.

Spicy Shrimp Tacos with Cilantro Lime Slaw

PREPARATION TIME: 15 min **COOKING TIME:** 5 min **MODE OF COOKING:** Sautéing

INGREDIENTS:

- ♥1 lb shrimp, peeled and deveined;
- ♥2 Tbsp taco seasoning;
- ♥1/4 cabbage, shredded;
- ♥1/4 cup cilantro, chopped;
- ♥2 limes, juiced;
- ♥1 Tbsp honey;
- ♥8 corn tortillas;
- ♥1 avocado, sliced;
- ♥1 Tbsp olive oil

DIRECTIONS: 1 Heat oil in a pan over medium heat; **2** Toss shrimp with taco seasoning and sauté until pink, about 3-4 min; **3** Mix cabbage, cilantro, lime juice, and honey for the slaw; **4** Warm tortillas; **5** Assemble tacos with shrimp, slaw, and avocado slices.

TIPS: 1 Add a dollop of sour cream for richness. **2** Use a grill pan for extra flavor.

N.V.: Calories: 290, Fat: 9g, Carbs: 32g, Protein: 23g, Sugar: 5g, Sodium: 480 mg, Potassium: 400 mg, Cholesterol: 120 mg, Glucose: 0 mg, Magnesium: 50 mg.

One-Pot Beef and Broccoli

PREPARATION TIME: 10 min **COOKING TIME:** 20 min **MODE OF COOKING:** Sautéing

INGREDIENTS:

- ♥1 lb beef sirloin, thinly sliced;
- ♥1 lb broccoli florets;
- ♥2 garlic cloves, minced;
- ♥1/4 cup soy sauce;
- ♥2 Tbsp cornstarch;
- ♥1 Tbsp olive oil;
- ♥1/2 cup beef broth;
- ♥1 Tbsp honey;
- ♥1 tsp ginger, grated

DIRECTIONS: 1 Heat oil in a large pan; **2** Brown beef slices, set aside; **3** In the same pan, add garlic and ginger, sauté for 1 min; **4** Add broccoli and broth, cover and simmer for 5 min; **5** Return beef to pan, add soy sauce and honey; **6** Dissolve cornstarch in a little water, add to pan to thicken sauce; **7** Cook until broccoli is tender and beef is coated with sauce.

TIPS: 1 Serve over steamed rice for a complete meal. **2** Sprinkle with sesame seeds before serving.

N.V.: Calories: 310, Fat: 10g, Carbs: 20g, Protein: 32g, Sugar: 6g, Sodium: 630 mg, Potassium: 640 mg, Cholesterol: 70 mg, Glucose: 0 mg, Magnesium: 42 mg.

Mushroom Risotto

PREPARATION TIME: 5 min **COOKING TIME:** 25 min **MODE OF COOKING:** Stirring

INGREDIENTS:

- ♥1 cup Arborio rice;
- ♥4 cups vegetable broth, heated;
- ♥1 lb mushrooms, sliced;
- ♥1 onion, finely chopped;
- ♥1/4 cup Parmesan cheese, grated;
- ♥2 Tbsp olive oil;
- ♥1/4 cup white wine;
- ♥Salt and pepper to taste

DIRECTIONS: 1 Heat oil in a large pan over medium heat; **2** Add onion, cook until translucent; **3** Add mushrooms, cook until browned; **4** Stir in rice to coat with oil; **5** Add wine, cook until absorbed; **6** Gradually add broth, stirring constantly, until rice is creamy and al dente; **7** Stir in Parmesan, season with salt and pepper.

TIPS: 1 Use a mix of wild mushrooms for depth of flavor. **2** Finish with a drizzle of truffle oil for a gourmet touch.

N.V.: Calories: 350, Fat: 12g, Carbs: 48g, Protein: 12g, Sugar: 3g, Sodium: 470 mg, Potassium: 300 mg, Cholesterol: 11 mg, Glucose: 0 mg, Magnesium: 20 mg.

Parmesan Herb Crusted Chicken

PREPARATION TIME: 10 min **COOKING TIME:** 20 min **MODE OF COOKING:** Baking

INGREDIENTS:

- ♥4 boneless chicken breasts;
- ♥1/2 cup grated Parmesan cheese;
- ♥1/4 cup breadcrumbs;
- ♥1 Tbsp dried Italian herbs;
- ♥2 Tbsp olive oil;
- ♥Salt and pepper to taste

DIRECTIONS: **1** Preheat oven to 375°F (190°C); **2** Combine Parmesan, breadcrumbs, herbs, salt, and pepper; **3** Brush chicken with olive oil; **4** Dredge in breadcrumb mixture; **5** Place on a greased baking sheet; **6** Bake for 20 min or until golden and cooked through.

TIPS: **1** Serve with a light arugula salad for a balanced meal. **2** For extra juiciness, brine the chicken for an hour before cooking.

N.V.: Calories: 330, Fat: 15g, Carbs: 9g, Protein: 38g, Sugar: 1g, Sodium: 390 mg, Potassium: 300 mg, Cholesterol: 95 mg, Glucose: 0 mg, Magnesium: 42 mg.

Vegetable Stir-Fry with Tofu

PREPARATION TIME: 10 min **COOKING TIME:** 10 min **MODE OF COOKING:** Stir-frying

INGREDIENTS:

- ♥1 lb tofu, cubed;
- ♥2 cups mixed vegetables (broccoli, bell peppers, carrots);
- ♥2 Tbsp soy sauce;
- ♥1 Tbsp sesame oil;
- ♥1 garlic clove, minced;
- ♥1 tsp ginger, grated;
- ♥1 Tbsp honey

DIRECTIONS: **1** Heat sesame oil in a large skillet over medium-high heat; **2** Add garlic and ginger, sauté for 1 min; **3** Add tofu and vegetables; **4** Stir-fry for 7-8 min; **5** Drizzle with soy sauce and honey; **6** Cook for an additional 2 min.

TIPS: **1** Press tofu before cooking to remove excess water and improve texture. **2** Add a splash of chili sauce for a spicy kick.

N.V.: Calories: 250, Fat: 12g, Carbs: 20g, Protein: 16g, Sugar: 7g, Sodium: 660 mg, Potassium: 400 mg, Cholesterol: 0 mg, Glucose: 0 mg, Magnesium: 60 mg.

Roasted Tomato and Basil Pasta

PREPARATION TIME: 10 min **COOKING TIME:** 25 min **MODE OF COOKING:** Roasting

INGREDIENTS:

- ♥2 cups cherry tomatoes;
- ♥3 cloves garlic, minced;
- ♥1/4 cup olive oil;
- ♥Salt and pepper to taste;
- ♥1 lb pasta;
- ♥1/2 cup fresh basil, chopped;
- ♥1/4 cup grated Parmesan cheese

DIRECTIONS: 1 Preheat oven to 400°F (204°C); **2** Toss tomatoes and garlic with olive oil, salt, and pepper; **3** Roast for 25 min until burst; **4** Cook pasta according to package instructions; **5** Toss pasta with roasted tomatoes and fresh basil; **6** Sprinkle with Parmesan before serving.

TIPS: 1 Use whole wheat pasta for added fiber. **2** Add red pepper flakes for a spicy twist.

N.V.: Calories: 410, Fat: 14g, Carbs: 60g, Protein: 13g, Sugar: 4g, Sodium: 190 mg, Potassium: 410 mg, Cholesterol: 4 mg, Glucose: 0 mg, Magnesium: 75 mg.

Balsamic Glazed Steak Rolls

PREPARATION TIME: 15 min **COOKING TIME:** 15 min **MODE OF COOKING:** Sautéing, Glazing

INGREDIENTS:

- ♥1 lb flank steak, thinly sliced;
- ♥1/2 cup balsamic vinegar;
- ♥1/4 cup honey;
- ♥2 carrots, julienned;
- ♥1 bell pepper, julienned;
- ♥1 zucchini, julienned;
- ♥Salt and pepper to taste;
- ♥1 Tbsp olive oil

DIRECTIONS: 1 Season steak slices with salt and pepper; **2** **3** Heat olive oil in a skillet over medium-high heat; **4** Sear steak rolls on all sides until browned, about 2 min per side; **5** Remove rolls and set aside; **6** Add balsamic vinegar and honey to the skillet, bring to a boil, reduce to a thick glaze; **7** Return steak rolls to the skillet, coat with glaze, and cook for an additional 2 min.

TIPS: 1 Secure steak rolls with toothpicks to keep them rolled while cooking. **2** Serve over a bed of mashed potatoes or rice to soak up the extra glaze.

N.V.: Calories: 310, Fat: 14g, Carbs: 18g, Protein: 28g, Sugar: 15g, Sodium: 220 mg, Potassium: 490 mg, Cholesterol: 70 mg, Glucose: 0 mg, Magnesium: 50 mg.

Creamy Lemon Chicken Piccata

PREPARATION TIME: 10 min **COOKING TIME:** 20 min **MODE OF COOKING:** Pan-frying

INGREDIENTS:

- ♥4 boneless chicken breasts, pounded thin;
- ♥1/4 cup flour;
- ♥2 Tbsp olive oil;
- ♥1/4 cup fresh lemon juice;
- ♥1/2 cup chicken broth;
- ♥1/4 cup capers;
- ♥1/4 cup heavy cream;
- ♥Salt and pepper to taste;
- ♥Parsley for garnish

DIRECTIONS: 1 Dredge chicken in flour seasoned with salt and pepper; **2** Heat oil in a pan over medium-high heat; **3** Cook chicken until golden and cooked through, about 4 min per side; **4** Remove chicken and set aside; **5** Add lemon juice, broth, and capers to the pan; **6** Bring to a boil and reduce by half; **7** Stir in cream, return chicken to the pan, and simmer for 5 min.

TIPS: 1 Garnish with chopped parsley for a fresh touch. **2** Serve with angel hair pasta to complement the creamy sauce.

N.V.: Calories: 295, Fat: 15g, Carbs: 8g, Protein: 30g, Sugar: 1g, Sodium: 530 mg, Potassium: 270 mg, Cholesterol: 85 mg, Glucose: 0 mg, Magnesium: 20 mg.

Spiced Lentil Stew with Kale

PREPARATION TIME: 10 min **COOKING TIME:** 25 min **MODE OF COOKING:** Simmering

INGREDIENTS:

- ♥1 cup dried lentils;
- ♥4 cups vegetable broth;
- ♥1 onion, diced;
- ♥2 carrots, diced;
- ♥2 cloves garlic, minced;
- ♥1 tsp ground cumin;
- ♥1 tsp curry powder;
- ♥2 cups kale, chopped;
- ♥Salt and pepper to taste;
- ♥1 Tbsp olive oil

DIRECTIONS: 1 Heat oil in a large pot over medium heat; **2** Add onion and garlic, sauté until translucent; **3** Stir in spices and cook for 1 min; **4** Add lentils, broth, and carrots; **5** Bring to a boil, reduce heat, and simmer until lentils are tender, about 20 min; **6** Stir in kale and cook until wilted, about 5 min.

TIPS: 1 Serve with a dollop of yogurt and a squeeze of lemon for extra flavor. **2** Add a pinch of chili flakes for a spicy kick.

N.V.: Calories: 265, Fat: 5g, Carbs: 40g, Protein: 18g, Sugar: 5g, Sodium: 590 mg, Potassium: 800 mg, Cholesterol: 0 mg, Glucose: 0 mg, Magnesium: 70 mg.

Baked Cod with Crispy Garlic Potatoes

PREPARATION TIME: 10 min **COOKING TIME:** 25 min **MODE OF COOKING:** Baking

INGREDIENTS:

- ♥4 cod fillets, 6 oz each;
- ♥1 lb small potatoes, halved;
- ♥4 cloves garlic, minced;
- ♥2 Tbsp olive oil;
- ♥1 lemon, sliced;
- ♥Salt and pepper to taste;
- ♥Parsley for garnish

DIRECTIONS: 1 Preheat oven to 400°F (204°C); **2** Toss potatoes with half the olive oil, garlic, salt, and pepper; **3** Spread on a baking tray and roast for 15 min; **4** Place cod on the tray, top with remaining oil and lemon slices; **5** Bake for 10 min until fish is cooked through.

TIPS: 1 Garnish with parsley before serving for a fresh look. **2** Ensure potatoes are cut uniformly for even cooking.

N.V.: Calories: 320, Fat: 10g, Carbs: 28g, Protein: 30g, Sugar: 2g, Sodium: 75 mg, Potassium: 950 mg, Cholesterol: 60 mg, Glucose: 0 mg, Magnesium: 85 mg.

Stuffed Bell Peppers with Quinoa and Black Beans

PREPARATION TIME: 15 min **COOKING TIME:** 30 min **MODE OF COOKING:** Baking

INGREDIENTS:

- ♥4 large bell peppers, tops cut, seeded;
- ♥1 cup quinoa, cooked;
- ♥1 can black beans, drained and rinsed;
- ♥1 cup corn;
- ♥1/2 cup tomato sauce;
- ♥1 tsp chili powder;
- ♥1/2 cup shredded Monterey Jack cheese;
- ♥Salt and pepper to taste

DIRECTIONS: 1 Preheat oven to 350°F (177°C); **2** Mix quinoa, black beans, corn, tomato sauce, chili powder, salt, and pepper in a bowl; **3** Stuff mixture into bell peppers; **4** Top with cheese; **5** Place in a baking dish and cover with foil; **6** Bake for 30 min, uncovering in the last 10 min.

TIPS: 1 Serve with a dollop of sour cream or guacamole. **2** Sprinkle with cilantro for an added fresh flavor.

N.V.: Calories: 285, Fat: 8g, Carbs: 42g, Protein: 14g, Sugar: 8g, Sodium: 480 mg, Potassium: 640 mg, Cholesterol: 15 mg, Glucose: 0 mg, Magnesium: 55 mg.

PREPARATION TIME: 10 min **COOKING TIME:** 20 min **MODE OF COOKING:** Simmering

INGREDIENTS:

- ♥1 lb chicken breast, cubed;
- ♥1 can coconut milk;
- ♥2 Tbsp green curry paste;
- ♥1 bag mixed Asian vegetables (broccoli, snap peas, carrots);
- ♥1 Tbsp fish sauce;
- ♥1 tsp sugar;
- ♥Basil leaves for garnish;
- ♥1 Tbsp vegetable oil

DIRECTIONS: 1 Heat oil in a large skillet over medium heat; **2** Add green curry paste, stir for 1 min; **3** Add chicken, cook until browned; **4** Pour in coconut milk, bring to a simmer; **5** Add vegetables, fish sauce, and sugar; **6** Cook for 10 min until vegetables are tender and chicken is cooked through.

TIPS: 1 Garnish with fresh basil leaves before serving. **2** Serve with jasmine rice to complement the flavors.

N.V.: Calories: 310, Fat: 18g, Carbs: 10g, Protein: 28g, Sugar: 5g, Sodium: 710 mg, Potassium: 650 mg, Cholesterol: 75 mg, Glucose: 0 mg, Magnesium: 60 mg.

7. SNACKS AND SIDES

In the symphony of a well-rounded meal, snacks and sides play more than just a supporting role; they bring harmony and highlight the main event, while sometimes, quite capably, standing out as stars on their own. This chapter delves into the art of crafting snacks and sides that not only complement your meals but also provide delightful bursts of flavor to invigorate your day, at any hour.

Imagine the gentle crunch of a perfectly roasted brussels sprout that contrasts sublimely with a tender main course, or the zesty lift a citrus-infused quinoa salad adds to your dinner. These are the touches that transform meals from routine to remarkable, ensuring that eating well remains both a pleasure and a breeze.

Each recipe here is designed with the dual purpose of ease and impact. Whether you're looking for a quick snack to stave off afternoon hunger or a side dish that will brighten up a family dinner, these culinary creations are crafted to be straightforward and satisfying. They are the perfect answer to the question of what to eat when you want something small yet mighty in flavor and nutrition.

From dips that make vegetables exciting again to grains brought to life with herbs and spices, each dish is a small testament to the fact that great things often come in simple packages. These snacks and sides are not only companions to your meals but also providers of balance and bursts of required nutrients, keeping you energized and content until the next meal.

As you explore these recipes, allow yourself the flexibility to mix and match, creating new mealtime traditions that speak directly to your needs and those of your family. Whether it's a mid-morning nibble or a side that steals the show, you'll find that these additions are just what you need to complete a plate and a day full of dietary success.

Roasted Chickpeas with Rosemary and Sea Salt

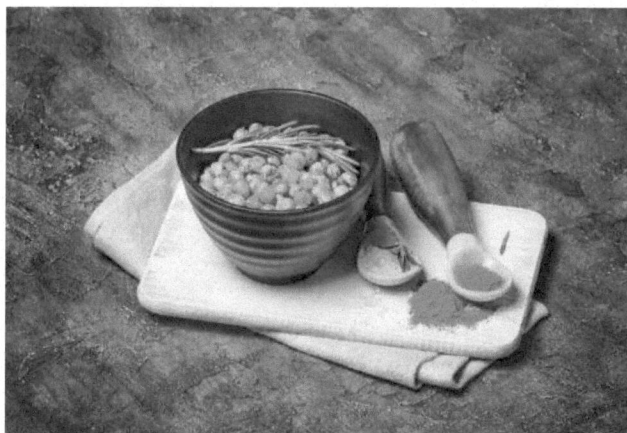

PREPARATION TIME: 5 min **COOKING TIME:** 30 min **MODE OF COOKING:** Roasting

INGREDIENTS:

- ♥2 cans chickpeas, drained and rinsed;
- ♥2 Tbsp olive oil;
- ♥1 Tbsp fresh rosemary, chopped;
- ♥Sea salt to taste

DIRECTIONS: 1 Preheat oven to 375°F (190°C); **2** Pat chickpeas dry with paper towels; **3** Toss with olive oil and rosemary; **4** Spread on a baking sheet; **5** Roast for 30 min, shaking the pan halfway through.

TIPS: 1 Ensure chickpeas are completely dry for maximum crispiness. **2** Great as a salad topping or healthy snack.

N.V.: Calories: 210, Fat: 10g, Carbs: 23g, Protein: 7g, Sugar: 4g, Sodium: 400 mg, Potassium: 290 mg, Cholesterol: 0 mg, Glucose: 0 mg, Magnesium: 48 mg.

Crispy Parmesan Garlic Edamame

PREPARATION TIME: 5 min **COOKING TIME:** 15 min **MODE OF COOKING:** Baking

INGREDIENTS:

- ♥2 cups frozen edamame, thawed;
- ♥2 Tbsp olive oil;
- ♥1/4 cup Parmesan cheese, grated;
- ♥3 cloves garlic, minced;
- ♥Salt and pepper to taste

DIRECTIONS: 1 Preheat oven to 400°F (204°C); **2** Toss edamame with olive oil, garlic, salt, and pepper; **3** Spread on a baking sheet; **4** Sprinkle with Parmesan cheese; **5** Bake for 15 min until crispy.

TIPS: 1 Serve warm for the best flavor and texture. **2** Sprinkle with red pepper flakes for a spicy kick.

N.V.: Calories: 190, Fat: 12g, Carbs: 10g, Protein: 12g, Sugar: 2g, Sodium: 180 mg, Potassium: 430 mg, Cholesterol: 4 mg, Glucose: 0 mg, Magnesium: 50 mg.

Sweet Potato Fries with Thyme

PREPARATION TIME: 10 min **COOKING TIME:** 25 min **MODE OF COOKING:** Baking

INGREDIENTS:

- ♥3 large sweet potatoes, peeled and cut into fries;
- ♥2 Tbsp olive oil;
- ♥1 Tbsp fresh thyme, minced;
- ♥Salt and pepper to taste

DIRECTIONS: 1 Preheat oven to 425°F (218°C); **2** Toss sweet potato fries with olive oil, thyme, salt, and pepper; **3** Spread in a single layer on a baking sheet; **4** Bake for 25 min, turning halfway through.

TIPS: 1 Serve with a side of Greek yogurt mixed with lime juice for dipping. **2** Space fries evenly to ensure they crisp up.

N.V.: Calories: 180, Fat: 7g, Carbs: 26g, Protein: 2g, Sugar: 5g, Sodium: 70 mg, Potassium: 440 mg, Cholesterol: 0 mg, Glucose: 0 mg, Magnesium: 30 mg.

Cucumber Dill Salad with Lemon Yogurt Dressing

PREPARATION TIME: 10 min **COOKING TIME:** 0 min **MODE OF COOKING:** Mixing

INGREDIENTS:

- ♥2 large cucumbers, thinly sliced;
- ♥1/2 cup plain Greek yogurt;
- ♥2 Tbsp lemon juice;
- ♥2 Tbsp fresh dill, chopped;
- ♥Salt and pepper to taste

DIRECTIONS: 1 In a large bowl, combine cucumbers and dill; **2** In a small bowl, whisk together yogurt, lemon juice, salt, and pepper; **3** Pour dressing over cucumbers and toss to coat.

TIPS: 1 Chill for at least 30 min before serving for enhanced flavors. **2** Add thinly sliced red onions for extra bite.

N.V.: Calories: 70, Fat: 1g, Carbs: 12g, Protein: 4g, Sugar: 6g, Sodium: 45 mg, Potassium: 187 mg, Cholesterol: 3 mg, Glucose: 0 mg, Magnesium: 24 mg.

Grilled Zucchini with Lemon Herb Vinaigrette

PREPARATION TIME: 10 min **COOKING TIME:** 10 min **MODE OF COOKING:** Grilling

INGREDIENTS:

- ♥4 medium zucchini, sliced lengthwise;
- ♥2 Tbsp olive oil;
- ♥1 lemon, juiced;
- ♥1 Tbsp fresh herbs (basil, parsley, thyme), chopped;
- ♥Salt and pepper to taste

DIRECTIONS: 1 Preheat grill to medium-high; **2** Brush zucchini slices with olive oil and season with salt and pepper; **3** Grill for about 5 min on each side or until tender; **4** Whisk together lemon juice, herbs, and additional olive oil; **5** Drizzle vinaigrette over grilled zucchini.

TIPS: 1 Perfect as a side or chopped into salads. **2** Vary the herbs based on availability or preference.

N.V.: Calories: 90, Fat: 7g, Carbs: 7g, Protein: 2g, Sugar: 4g, Sodium: 10 mg, Potassium: 510 mg, Cholesterol: 0 mg, Glucose: 0 mg, Magnesium: 30 mg.

Maple Cinnamon Roasted Chickpeas

PREPARATION TIME: 5 min **COOKING TIME:** 30 min **MODE OF COOKING:** Roasting

INGREDIENTS:

- ♥2 cans chickpeas, drained, rinsed, and dried;
- ♥1 Tbsp olive oil;
- ♥2 Tbsp maple syrup;
- ♥1 tsp ground cinnamon;
- ♥1/4 tsp salt

DIRECTIONS: 1 Preheat oven to 375°F (190°C); **2** Toss chickpeas with olive oil, maple syrup, cinnamon, and salt; **3** Spread on a baking sheet in a single layer; **4** Roast for 30 min, stirring halfway through, until crispy.

TIPS: 1 Let chickpeas cool completely on the tray to enhance crispiness. **2** Store in an airtight container to maintain crunch.

N.V.: Calories: 210, Fat: 6g, Carbs: 30g, Protein: 7g, Sugar: 8g, Sodium: 300 mg, Potassium: 332 mg, Cholesterol: 0 mg, Glucose: 0 mg, Magnesium: 48 mg.

Spicy Lime Edamame

PREPARATION TIME: 2 min **COOKING TIME:** 5 min **MODE OF COOKING:** Boiling

INGREDIENTS:

- ♥2 cups frozen edamame;
- ♥1 lime, juiced;
- ♥1/2 tsp chili powder;
- ♥1/4 tsp salt

DIRECTIONS: 1 Boil edamame in salted water for 5 min; **2** Drain and toss with lime juice, chili powder, and salt.

TIPS: 1 Serve warm for a zesty snack. **2** Perfect pairing with a cold beverage.

N.V.: Calories: 120, Fat: 5g, Carbs: 10g, Protein: 12g, Sugar: 2g, Sodium: 240 mg, Potassium: 482 mg, Cholesterol: 0 mg, Glucose: 0 mg, Magnesium: 50 mg.

Garlic Parmesan Kale Chips

PREPARATION TIME: 5 min **COOKING TIME:** 10 min **MODE OF COOKING:** Baking

INGREDIENTS:

- ♥1 bunch kale, washed and torn into pieces;
- ♥1 Tbsp olive oil;
- ♥1/4 cup grated Parmesan cheese;
- ♥1 garlic clove, minced;
- ♥Salt to taste

DIRECTIONS: 1 Preheat oven to 350°F (177°C); **2** Toss kale with olive oil, garlic, and salt; **3** Spread on a baking sheet; **4** Sprinkle with Parmesan; **5** Bake for 10 min until crisp.

TIPS: 1 Ensure kale is dry before oiling for the crispiest results. **2** Watch closely to prevent burning.

N.V.: Calories: 150, Fat: 9g, Carbs: 10g, Protein: 8g, Sugar: 0g, Sodium: 250 mg, Potassium: 447 mg, Cholesterol: 11 mg, Glucose: 0 mg, Magnesium: 30 mg.

Baked Sweet Potato Wedges

PREPARATION TIME: 10 min **COOKING TIME:** 25 min **MODE OF COOKING:** Baking
INGREDIENTS:
- ♥3 large sweet potatoes, cut into wedges;
- ♥2 Tbsp olive oil;
- ♥1 tsp smoked paprika;
- ♥Salt and pepper to taste

DIRECTIONS: 1 Preheat oven to 400°F (204°C); **2** Toss sweet potato wedges with olive oil, paprika, salt, and pepper; **3** Spread in a single layer on a baking sheet; **4** Bake for 25 min until tender and crispy.

TIPS: 1 Serve with a yogurt-based dip for added flavor. **2** Sprinkle with fresh herbs like thyme before serving.

N.V.: Calories: 180, Fat: 7g, Carbs: 27g, Protein: 2g, Sugar: 5g, Sodium: 150 mg, Potassium: 474 mg, Cholesterol: 0 mg, Glucose: 0 mg, Magnesium: 30 mg.

Zesty Quinoa Salad

PREPARATION TIME: 5 min **COOKING TIME:** 15 min **MODE OF COOKING:** Boiling
INGREDIENTS:
- ♥1 cup quinoa, rinsed;
- ♥2 cups water;
- ♥1/2 cucumber, diced;
- ♥1 bell pepper, diced;

♥1/4 cup feta cheese, crumbled;

♥1/4 cup lemon juice;

♥2 Tbsp olive oil;

♥Salt and pepper to taste

DIRECTIONS: 1 Boil quinoa in water until fluffy, about 15 min; **2** Cool slightly; **3** Mix with cucumber, bell pepper, and feta; **4** Dress with lemon juice, olive oil, salt, and pepper.

TIPS: 1 Chill before serving to enhance flavors. **2** Add fresh herbs like parsley or mint for extra freshness.

N.V.: Calories: 245, Fat: 10g, Carbs: 32g, Protein: 8g, Sugar: 2g, Sodium: 180 mg, Potassium: 320 mg, Cholesterol: 8 mg, Glucose: 0 mg, Magnesium: 64 mg.

Roasted Brussels Sprouts with Balsamic Glaze

PREPARATION TIME: 5 min **COOKING TIME:** 20 min **MODE OF COOKING:** Roasting

INGREDIENTS:

♥2 cups Brussels sprouts, halved;

♥2 Tbsp olive oil;

♥Salt and pepper to taste;

♥2 Tbsp balsamic vinegar;

♥1 Tbsp honey

DIRECTIONS: 1 Preheat oven to 400°F (204°C); **2** Toss Brussels sprouts with olive oil, salt, and pepper; **3** Roast for 20 min, turning halfway; **4** Drizzle with a mixture of balsamic vinegar and honey in the last 5 min.

TIPS: 1 The glaze adds a nice sheen and a punch of flavor. **2** Perfect as a holiday side dish.

N.V.: Calories: 140, Fat: 7g, Carbs: 17g, Protein: 3g, Sugar: 7g, Sodium: 25 mg, Potassium: 441 mg, Cholesterol: 0 mg, Glucose: 0 mg, Magnesium: 22 mg.

Cauliflower Tots

PREPARATION TIME: 15 min **COOKING TIME:** 20 min **MODE OF COOKING:** Baking

INGREDIENTS:

♥1 large cauliflower, grated;

♥1 egg, beaten;

♥1/4 cup breadcrumbs;

♥1/4 cup grated Parmesan cheese;

♥1 tsp garlic powder;

♥Salt and pepper to taste

DIRECTIONS: 1 Preheat oven to 375°F (190°C); **2** Steam grated cauliflower for 5 min; **3** Squeeze out excess moisture; **4** Mix with egg, breadcrumbs, Parmesan, garlic powder, salt, and pepper; **5** Shape into tots; **6** Bake for 20 min, turning halfway.

TIPS: 1 Serve with a side of marinara sauce for dipping. **2** Ensure all water is squeezed from cauliflower to keep tots crispy.

N.V.: Calories: 100, Fat: 4g, Carbs: 10g, Protein: 7g, Sugar: 2g, Sodium: 200 mg, Potassium: 320 mg, Cholesterol: 30 mg, Glucose: 0 mg, Magnesium: 20 mg.

Stuffed Mushrooms with Spinach and Cream Cheese

PREPARATION TIME: 10 min **COOKING TIME:** 20 min **MODE OF COOKING:** Baking

INGREDIENTS:

♥12 large mushroom caps, stems removed;

♥1 cup spinach, chopped;

♥1/2 cup cream cheese, softened;

♥1/4 cup breadcrumbs;

♥2 cloves garlic, minced;

♥Salt and pepper to taste;

♥2 Tbsp olive oil

DIRECTIONS: 1 Preheat oven to 375°F (190°C); **2** Sauté spinach and garlic in 1 Tbsp olive oil until spinach is wilted; **3** Mix spinach with cream cheese, breadcrumbs, salt, and pepper; **4** Stuff mixture into mushroom caps; **5** Drizzle with remaining olive oil; **6** Bake for 20 min.

TIPS: 1 Perfect for parties as a fancy yet easy appetizer. **2** Experiment with different types of cheese for varied flavors.

N.V.: Calories: 150, Fat: 10g, Carbs: 9g, Protein: 5g, Sugar: 2g, Sodium: 180 mg, Potassium: 300 mg, Cholesterol: 22 mg, Glucose: 0 mg, Magnesium: 15 mg.

Greek Yogurt Dip with Fresh Herbs

PREPARATION TIME: 5 min **COOKING TIME:** 0 min **MODE OF COOKING:** Mixing

INGREDIENTS:

♥1 cup Greek yogurt;

♥1/4 cup chopped fresh herbs (dill, parsley, chives);

♥1 lemon, zested and juiced;

♥1 clove garlic, minced;

♥Salt and pepper to taste

DIRECTIONS: 1 Combine all ingredients in a bowl; **2** Mix until well blended; **3** Chill before serving to let flavors meld.

TIPS: 1 Serve with vegetable sticks or whole grain crackers. **2** Can be used as a healthy sandwich spread.

N.V.: Calories: 60, Fat: 1g, Carbs: 5g, Protein: 9g, Sugar: 3g, Sodium: 45 mg, Potassium: 120 mg, Cholesterol: 5 mg, Glucose: 0 mg, Magnesium: 15 mg.

8. DESSERTS AND TREATS

Embarking on a journey of healthy eating doesn't mean saying goodbye to desserts. Quite the contrary—it's about redefining what treats can and should look like to fit into a lifestyle that values well-being and satisfaction equally. In this chapter, we explore how to indulge wisely, crafting desserts that delight the taste buds without derailing your health goals.

Imagine transforming the ripe, lush fruits of the season into a vibrant berry compote, or whipping up a chocolate mousse that's as airy and rich as it is nourishing. Here, desserts aren't just the finale to a meal; they are a celebration of flavors, made with ingredients that serve your body well. We focus on natural sweeteners, whole grains, and fresh fruits to create sweets that you can savor without guilt.

Think of a lemon tart with a crust made from ground almonds and a filling that's zesty and subtly sweet, or a peach crumble where the natural sweetness of the fruit sings through a crunchy topping spiced just right. These desserts are not only a treat for the palate but are also easy to assemble, ensuring that even the busiest among us can enjoy a touch of sweetness in our lives.

This approach to desserts is about balance and creativity. It's about looking at what we traditionally consider indulgent and asking how it can be better aligned with a nourishing lifestyle. Each recipe in this chapter is designed not only to satisfy your sweet tooth but also to contribute to your health, using ingredients that enhance rather than compromise your well-being.

So, let us put aside any notions that healthy eating must be devoid of the joy of a good dessert. Let's embrace a new perspective, where every sweet bite is as good for the body as it is delightful to the soul. After all, a life without treats isn't very sweet at all, and here, we find the perfect blend of health, happiness, and indulgence.

BAKED APPLE WITH CINNAMON AND NUTS

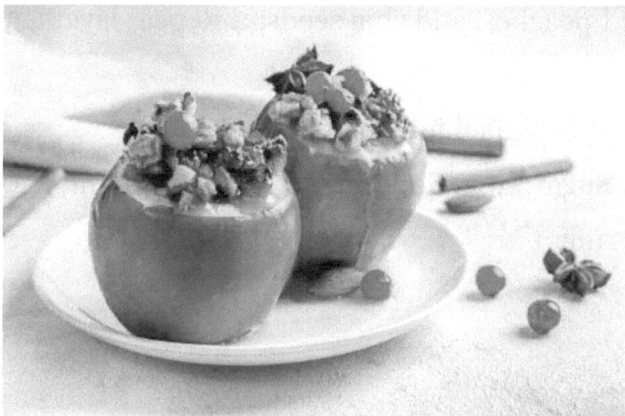

PREPARATION TIME: 10 min **COOKING TIME:** 20 min **MODE OF COOKING:** Baking
INGREDIENTS:
- ♥4 large apples, cored;
- ♥4 tsp honey;
- ♥1/2 tsp ground cinnamon;
- ♥1/4 cup walnuts, chopped **DIRECTIONS: 1** Place cored apples on a baking dish; **2** Drizzle each apple with 1 tsp honey and sprinkle with cinnamon; **3** Top with chopped walnuts; **4** Bake at 375°F

(190°C) until apples are soft. **TIPS:** **1** Serve warm with a dollop of Greek yogurt; **2** Sprinkle with ground flaxseed for added omega-3s. **N.V.:** Calories: 190, Fat: 5g, Carbs: 36g, Protein: 2g, Sugar: 30g, Sodium: 2 mg, Potassium: 195 mg, Cholesterol: 0 mg, Glucose: 0 mg, Magnesium: 20 mg.

CHOCOLATE AVOCADO MOUSSE

PREPARATION TIME: 15 min **COOKING TIME:** 0 min **MODE OF COOKING:** Blending

INGREDIENTS:

- ♥2 ripe avocados;
- ♥1/4 cup coca polder;
- ♥1/4 cup honey;
- ♥1 tsp vanilla extract;
- ♥Pinch of salt

DIRECTIONS: **1** Blend all ingredients until smooth; **2** Chill in the refrigerator for at least 1 hr before serving.

TIPS: **1** Top with fresh raspberries; **2** Add a sprinkle of chia seeds for extra fiber.

N.V.: Calories: 240, Fat: 15g, Carbs: 28g, Protein: 3g, Sugar: 17g, Sodium: 5 mg, Potassium: 487 mg, Cholesterol: 0 mg, Glucose: 0 mg, Magnesium: 30 mg.

PEACH AND CHIA SEED PARFAIT

PREPARATION TIME: 10 min **COOKING TIME:** 0 min **MODE OF COOKING:** Layering

INGREDIENTS:

- ♥1 cup Greek yogurt, unsweetened;
- ♥2 peaches, sliced;
- ♥2 Tbsp chia seeds;
- ♥1 tsp honey

DIRECTIONS: **1** In a glass, layer Greek yogurt, sliced peaches, and chia seeds; **2** Repeat layers; **3** Drizzle honey on top before serving.

TIPS: **1** Substitute peaches with any seasonal fruit; **2** Serve chilled for best flavor.

N.V.: Calories: 215, Fat: 3g, Carbs: 34g, Protein: 14g, Sugar: 28g, Sodium: 50 mg, Potassium: 350 mg, Cholesterol: 10 mg, Glucose: 0 mg, Magnesium: 55 mg.

RICOTTA AND BERRY COMPOTE

PREPARATION TIME: 5 min **COOKING TIME:** 15 min **MODE OF COOKING:** Simmering

INGREDIENTS:

- ♥1 cup fresh berries (mixed);
- ♥1 cup ricotta cheese;
- ♥2 Tbsp honey;
- ♥1/2 tsp lemon zest

DIRECTIONS: 1 Simmer berries with honey and lemon zest over medium heat until syrupy; **2** Let cool slightly; **3** Serve over ricotta cheese.

TIPS: 1 Use part-skim ricotta to reduce fat content; **2** Garnish with mint for a fresh flavor.

N.V.: Calories: 180, Fat: 8g, Carbs: 18g, Protein: 10g, Sugar: 16g, Sodium: 80 mg, Potassium: 90 mg, Cholesterol: 35 mg, Glucose: 0 mg, Magnesium: 20 mg.

ALMOND AND DATE TRUFFLES

PREPARATION TIME: 20 min **COOKING TIME:** 0 min **MODE OF COOKING:** Mixing

INGREDIENTS:

- ♥1 cup dates, pitted;
- ♥1/2 cup almonds;
- ♥1/4 cup shredded coconut, unsweetened;
- ♥1 tsp vanilla extract

DIRECTIONS: 1 Process dates and almonds in a food processor until finely chopped; **2** Add vanilla extract and form into balls; **3** Roll balls in shredded coconut.

TIPS: 1 Keep truffles chilled in the refrigerator; **2** Roll truffles in cocoa powder for a chocolate version.

N.V.: Calories: 130, Fat: 7g, Carbs: 16g, Protein: 2g, Sugar: 12g, Sodium: 2 mg, Potassium: 210 mg, Cholesterol: 0 mg, Glucose: 0 mg, Magnesium: 35 mg.

GRILLED PINEAPPLE WITH HONEY AND CINNAMON

PREPARATION TIME: 10 min **COOKING TIME:** 10 min **MODE OF COOKING:** Grilling

INGREDIENTS:

- ♥1 pineapple, peeled and cored, cut into rings;
- ♥1 Tbsp honey;
- ♥1/2 tsp cinnamon

DIRECTIONS: 1 Grill pineapple rings over medium heat until char marks appear; **2** Whisk together honey and cinnamon; **3** Brush over pineapple while hot.

TIPS: 1 Serve with a scoop of low-fat vanilla ice cream; **2** Sprinkle with toasted coconut flakes.

N.V.: Calories: 100, Fat: 0g, Carbs: 25g, Protein: 1g, Sugar: 20g, Sodium: 1 mg, Potassium: 120 mg, Cholesterol: 0 mg, Glucose: 0 mg, Magnesium: 10 mg.

SPICED CARROT CAKE BARS

PREPARATION TIME: 15 min **COOKING TIME:** 30 min **MODE OF COOKING:** Baking

INGREDIENTS:

- ♥2 cups grated carrots;
- ♥1 cup whole wheat flour;
- ♥1/2 cup applesauce, unsweetened;
- ♥1/4 cup honey;
- ♥2 eggs;
- ♥1 tsp baking powder;
- ♥1/2 tsp cinnamon;
- ♥1/4 tsp nutmeg

DIRECTIONS: 1 Mix all ingredients until well combined; **2** Pour into a lined baking pan; **3** Bake at 350°F (177°C) until a toothpick inserted comes out clean.

TIPS: 1 Frost with a blend of cream cheese and honey; **2** Add walnuts for extra crunch.

N.V.: Calories: 150, Fat: 3g, Carbs: 28g, Protein: 4g, Sugar: 15g, Sodium: 125 mg, Potassium: 180 mg, Cholesterol: 40 mg, Glucose: 0 mg, Magnesium: 20 mg.

GINGER PEAR SORBET

PREPARATION TIME: 15 min **COOKING TIME:** 0 min **MODE OF COOKING:** Freezing

INGREDIENTS:

- ♥3 ripe pears, peeled and cored;
- ♥1 Tbsp fresh ginger, grated;
- ♥Juice of 1 lemon;
- ♥2 Tbsp honey

DIRECTIONS: 1 Puree pears, ginger, lemon juice, and honey in a blender until smooth; **2** Freeze in an ice cream maker according to manufacturer's instructions, or place in a freezer-safe container and stir every 30 min until set.

TIPS: **1** Serve with a mint leaf garnish; **2** Add a splash of sparkling water when serving for a refreshing twist.

N.V.: Calories: 120, Fat: 0g, Carbs: 31g, Protein: 1g, Sugar: 25g, Sodium: 2 mg, Potassium: 150 mg, Cholesterol: 0 mg, Glucose: 0 mg, Magnesium: 10 mg.

BANANA CINNAMON ICE CREAM

PREPARATION TIME: 10 min **COOKING TIME:** 0 min **MODE OF COOKING:** Freezing

INGREDIENTS:
- ♥4 ripe bananas, sliced and frozen;
- ♥1/2 tsp cinnamon;
- ♥2 Tbsp almond milk;
- ♥1 tsp vanilla extract

DIRECTIONS: 1 Blend frozen bananas, cinnamon, almond milk, and vanilla in a food processor until creamy; **2** Freeze for an additional hour or serve immediately for a soft-serve texture.

TIPS: 1 Mix in dark chocolate chips for added indulgence; **2** Top with chopped nuts for a crunchy texture.

N.V.: Calories: 110, Fat: 1g, Carbs: 27g, Protein: 1g, Sugar: 14g, Sodium: 3 mg, Potassium: 422 mg, Cholesterol: 0 mg, Glucose: 0 mg, Magnesium: 27 mg.

AVOCADO LIME CHEESECAKE

PREPARATION TIME: 20 min **COOKING TIME:** 0 min **MODE OF COOKING:** Chilling

INGREDIENTS:
- ♥1 ripe avocado;
- ♥1/2 cup cashews, soaked for 4 hours and drained;
- ♥1/4 cup lime juice;
- ♥1/4 cup honey;
- ♥1 tsp vanilla extract;
- ♥1/2 cup coconut oil, melted

DIRECTIONS: 1 Blend avocado, cashews, lime juice, honey, vanilla, and coconut oil until smooth; **2** Pour into a prepared crust and chill until set, about 2 hours.

TIPS: 1 Use a crust made from ground almonds and dates; **2** Garnish with lime zest before serving.

N.V.: Calories: 300, Fat: 25g, Carbs: 20g, Protein: 3g, Sugar: 15g, Sodium: 7 mg, Potassium: 290 mg, Cholesterol: 0 mg, Glucose: 0 mg, Magnesium: 50 mg.

RASPBERRY ALMOND THUMBPRINT COOKIES

PREPARATION TIME: 15 min **COOKING TIME:** 10 min **MODE OF COOKING:** Baking

INGREDIENTS:

- ♥1 cup almond flour;
- ♥1/4 cup coconut oil, softened;
- ♥1/4 cup honey;
- ♥1 tsp vanilla extract;
- ♥Raspberry jam, unsweetened

DIRECTIONS: 1 Mix almond flour, coconut oil, honey, and vanilla to form a dough; **2** Shape into balls, press a thumbprint into each, fill with a small spoonful of jam; **3** Bake at 350°F (177°C) for 10 min.

TIPS: 1 Use any sugar-free jam as an alternative; **2** Sprinkle with powdered erythritol for a snowy effect.

N.V.: Calories: 130, Fat: 9g, Carbs: 11g, Protein: 3g, Sugar: 7g, Sodium: 2 mg, Potassium: 10 mg, Cholesterol: 0 mg, Glucose: 0 mg, Magnesium: 40 mg.

COCONUT MILK RICE PUDDING

PREPARATION TIME: 5 min **COOKING TIME:** 25 min **MODE OF COOKING:** Simmering

INGREDIENTS:

- ♥1/2 cup arborio rice;
- ♥1 can coconut milk;
- ♥1/4 cup honey;
- ♥1/2 tsp vanilla extract;
- ♥Pinch of salt

DIRECTIONS: 1 Combine all ingredients in a saucepan; **2** Bring to a simmer, stirring frequently, until rice is tender and creamy, about 25 min.

TIPS: 1 Top with a sprinkle of cinnamon; **2** Add raisins during the last 5 min of cooking for added sweetness.

N.V.: Calories: 215, Fat: 8g, Carbs: 34g, Protein: 3g, Sugar: 12g, Sodium: 15 mg, Potassium: 30 mg, Cholesterol: 0 mg, Glucose: 0 mg, Magnesium: 15 mg.

PUMPKIN SPICE BARS

PREPARATION TIME: 10 min **COOKING TIME:** 20 min **MODE OF COOKING:** Baking

INGREDIENTS:

- ♥2 cups pumpkin puree;

♥1/2 cup almond flour;

♥1/4 cup honey;

♥2 eggs;

♥1 tsp pumpkin pie spice;

♥1/4 tsp salt

DIRECTIONS: 1 Mix all ingredients until well blended; **2** Pour into a lined baking pan; **3** Bake at 350°F (177°C) until set, about 20 min.

TIPS: 1 Cool completely and cut into bars; **2** Drizzle with a glaze made from Greek yogurt and honey.

N.V.: Calories: 150, Fat: 7g, Carbs: 18g, Protein: 5g, Sugar: 10g, Sodium: 55 mg, Potassium: 90 mg, Cholesterol: 40 mg, Glucose: 0 mg, Magnesium: 30 mg.

HONEY LEMON GELATO

PREPARATION TIME: 10 min **COOKING TIME:** 0 min **MODE OF COOKING:** Freezing

INGREDIENTS:

♥2 cups Greek yogurt, unsweetened;

♥1/4 cup honey;

♥1/4 cup lemon juice;

♥1 Tbsp lemon zest

DIRECTIONS: 1 Whisk together yogurt, honey, lemon juice, and zest until smooth; **2** Freeze in an ice cream maker or stir every 30 min in a freezer until set.

TIPS: 1 Serve immediately for a soft serve texture; **2** Garnish with fresh mint leaves.

N.V.: Calories: 130, Fat: 3g, Carbs: 20g, Protein: 8g, Sugar: 18g, Sodium: 35 mg, Potassium: 90 mg, Cholesterol: 10 mg, Glucose: 0 mg, Magnesium: 15 mg.

9. Drinks and Beverages

Step into a refreshing chapter where we celebrate the power of drinks and beverages to enhance our health and brighten our days. Here, we embark on a flavorful journey that brings both nourishment and delight with each sip. Whether it's starting the morning with a vibrant smoothie, enjoying a hydrating midday sip, or unwinding in the evening with a soothing herbal tea, this chapter is dedicated to drinks that do more than quench thirst—they invigorate and heal.

Imagine the joy of blending fresh fruits with leafy greens to create a smoothie that's not only a feast for the eyes but a fountain of vitamins and minerals. Or the ritual of steeping carefully chosen herbs to brew a tea that calms and centers the mind. In this chapter, each recipe is crafted to support your health goals, from boosting immunity to enhancing digestion, all while keeping your taste buds engaged.

Drinks and beverages hold a unique place in our diet. They can be transformative, serving as both healers and hydrators, energizers and soothers. They often play a background role in our meals, but here, they take center stage, showing that what we drink is just as important as what we eat. With an emphasis on fresh ingredients, minimal added sugars, and lots of flavor, these drinks are designed to fit seamlessly into a healthy lifestyle, aligning with the principles of the DASH diet to support heart health and overall well-being.

From homemade almond milk that serves as a creamy base for a variety of concoctions to a ginger turmeric shot that provides an anti-inflammatory boost, the beverages in this chapter are both creative and health-conscious. Each drink is an opportunity to experiment with natural flavors and to enjoy the health benefits that come from nature's bounty.

This chapter is not just a collection of recipes; it's an invitation to explore, to taste, and to transform your drinking habits into a joyful, health-enhancing element of your daily routine. So, grab your blender, kettle, or shaker—delicious, healthful hydration awaits.

CUCUMBER MINT REFRESHER

PREPARATION TIME: 5 min **COOKING TIME:** 0 min **MODE OF COOKING:** Blending

INGREDIENTS:

- ♥1 large cucumber, peeled;
- ♥8 mint leaves;
- ♥Juice of 1 lime;
- ♥1 tsp honey;
- ♥2 cups water

DIRECTIONS: 1 Blend all ingredients until smooth; **2** Strain and serve chilled.

TIPS: 1 Add sparkling water for a fizzy variation; **2** Garnish with a slice of lime or cucumber. **N.V.:** Calories: 50, Fat: 0g, Carbs: 12g, Protein: 1g, Sugar: 10g, Sodium: 2 mg, Potassium: 187 mg, Cholesterol: 0 mg, Glucose: 0 mg, Magnesium: 14 mg.

GINGER TURMERIC TEA

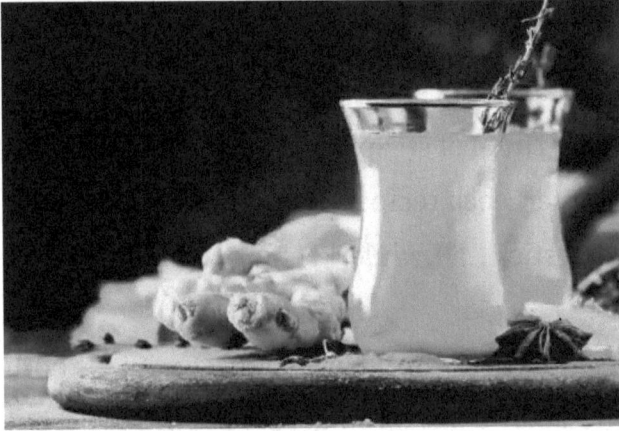

PREPARATION TIME: 5 min **COOKING TIME:** 10 min **MODE OF COOKING:** Simmering

INGREDIENTS:

- ♥1 inch ginger root, sliced;
- ♥1/2 tsp turmeric powder;
- ♥1 Tbsp honey;
- ♥4 cups water

DIRECTIONS: 1 Simmer ginger and turmeric in water for 10 min; **2** Strain, stir in honey, and serve.

TIPS: 1 Add a pinch of black pepper to increase curcumin absorption; **2** Serve with a lemon slice for extra zest.

N.V.: Calories: 40, Fat: 0g, Carbs: 10g, Protein: 0g, Sugar: 9g, Sodium: 10 mg, Potassium: 50 mg, Cholesterol: 0 mg, Glucose: 0 mg, Magnesium: 5 mg.

BLUEBERRY LAVENDER SMOOTHIE

PREPARATION TIME: 5 min **COOKING TIME:** 0 min **MODE OF COOKING:** Blending

INGREDIENTS:

- ♥1 cup blueberries;
- ♥1/2 cup Greek yogurt;
- ♥2 tsp dried lavender;
- ♥1 Tbsp honey;
- ♥1 cup almond milk

DIRECTIONS: 1 Blend all ingredients until smooth; **2** Serve immediately.

TIPS: 1 Freeze the blueberries for a thicker texture; **2** If lavender flavor is too strong, reduce to 1 tsp.

N.V.: Calories: 180, Fat: 3g, Carbs: 32g, Protein: 8g, Sugar: 25g, Sodium: 80 mg, Potassium: 90 mg, Cholesterol: 5 mg, Glucose: 0 mg, Magnesium: 20 mg.

CARROT GINGER ZINGER JUICE

PREPARATION TIME: 10 min **COOKING TIME:** 0 min **MODE OF COOKING:** Juicing

INGREDIENTS:

- ♥5 carrots, peeled;
- ♥1 apple, cored;
- ♥1 inch ginger root;
- ♥1/2 lemon, juiced

DIRECTIONS: 1 Juice all ingredients, stir and serve immediately.

TIPS: 1 Add a stalk of celery for extra nutrients; **2** Serve over ice for extra refreshment.

N.V.: Calories: 120, Fat: 1g, Carbs: 29g, Protein: 2g, Sugar: 21g, Sodium: 70 mg, Potassium: 690 mg, Cholesterol: 0 mg, Glucose: 0 mg, Magnesium: 30 mg.

PEACH BASIL ICED TEA

PREPARATION TIME: 15 min **COOKING TIME:** 5 min **MODE OF COOKING:** Steeping

INGREDIENTS:

- ♥4 black tea bags;
- ♥2 peaches, sliced;
- ♥10 basil leaves;
- ♥4 cups boiling water;
- ♥1 Tbsp honey

DIRECTIONS: 1 Steep tea bags, peach slices, and basil in boiling water for 5 min; **2** Remove tea bags, cool, and stir in honey; **3** Serve over ice.

TIPS: 1 Crush basil leaves slightly to release flavor; **2** Use ripe, juicy peaches for best taste.

N.V.: Calories: 30, Fat: 0g, Carbs: 8g, Protein: 1g, Sugar: 7g, Sodium: 0 mg, Potassium: 90 mg, Cholesterol: 0 mg, Glucose: 0 mg, Magnesium: 5 mg.

ALMOND MILK CHAI LATTE

PREPARATION TIME: 5 min **COOKING TIME:** 10 min **MODE OF COOKING:** Simmering

INGREDIENTS:

- ♥2 chai tea bags;
- ♥2 cups almond milk;
- ♥1 Tbsp honey;
- ♥1/2 tsp vanilla extract;
- ♥Cinnamon, for garnish

DIRECTIONS: 1 Heat almond milk until just simmering; **2** Add tea bags and steep for 5 min; **3** Remove tea bags, stir in honey and vanilla, serve hot with a sprinkle of cinnamon.

TIPS: 1 Froth the milk for a creamier texture; **2** Add a pinch of cardamom for extra spice.

N.V.: Calories: 100, Fat: 3g, Carbs: 16g, Protein: 2g, Sugar: 14g, Sodium: 100 mg, Potassium: 150 mg, Cholesterol: 0 mg, Glucose: 0 mg, Magnesium: 30 mg.

WATERMELON CUCUMBER COOLER

PREPARATION TIME: 10 min **COOKING TIME:** 0 min **MODE OF COOKING:** Blending

INGREDIENTS:

- ♥2 cups watermelon, cubed;
- ♥1/2 cucumber, peeled and cubed;
- ♥Juice of 1 lime;
- ♥1 Tbsp mint leaves;
- ♥1 cup ice

DIRECTIONS: 1 Blend watermelon, cucumber, lime juice, and mint until smooth; **2** Serve over ice.

TIPS: 1 Strain the mixture for a clearer juice; **2** Add a splash of sparkling water for fizz.

N.V.: Calories: 50, Fat: 0g, Carbs: 13g, Protein: 1g, Sugar: 10g, Sodium: 2 mg, Potassium: 180 mg, Cholesterol: 0 mg, Glucose: 0 mg, Magnesium: 15 mg.

10. Special Occasions and Entertaining

In the realm of home entertaining, food transforms from mere sustenance into a vibrant expression of culture, hospitality, and connection. Special occasions and gatherings call for dishes that not only nourish but also delight, impress, and bring people together. This chapter is a celebration of those moments—whether it's a festive holiday feast, a cozy family reunion, or an elegant dinner party. Here, we'll explore how to host with heart and health in mind, ensuring every guest leaves with a smile.

Imagine the warmth of a kitchen filled with the aromas of spiced, roasted vegetables and the comforting simmer of a low-sodium stew, ready to welcome friends on a chilly evening. Or consider the joy of laying out a summer spread of vibrant salads and fresh, grilled seafood, each dish telling a story of seasonal bounty and culinary craft. In this chapter, we intertwine the art of cooking with the joy of sharing, showing that a well-prepared meal can be the centerpiece of memorable gatherings.

Every recipe here is designed not only to meet the dietary guidelines of the DASH diet but to elevate them into something extraordinary. We focus on whole, unprocessed ingredients, mindful seasoning, and creative presentations that showcase that health-focused meals need not be mundane. From appetizers that tease the palate to desserts that satisfy the sweetest tooth without overindulgence, these dishes are crafted to impress without stress.

Hosting should be a pleasure, not a chore. Thus, this chapter also includes tips on how to prepare dishes ahead of time, how to set a table that speaks to the occasion, and how to manage portions and dietary preferences with grace and care. The art of entertaining is not just about the food—it's about the atmosphere, the conversation, and the shared experience.

So, whether you are planning a quiet anniversary dinner for two or a boisterous family gathering, let these recipes and tips guide you to create occasions that are healthy, happy, and unforgettable. After all, the heart of entertaining is not just to feed but to enrich—to offer food that fortifies the body, conversation that stimulates the mind, and hospitality that warms the heart.

ROASTED BRUSSELS SPROUTS WITH POMEGRANATE GLAZE

PREPARATION TIME: 10 min **COOKING TIME:** 20 min **MODE OF COOKING:** Roasting

INGREDIENTS:

- ♥1 lb Brussels sprouts, halved;
- ♥1 Tbsp olive oil;
- ♥1/4 cup pomegranate molasses;

♥Salt and pepper to taste

DIRECTIONS: **1** Toss Brussels sprouts with olive oil, salt, and pepper; **2** Roast at 400°F (204°C) until crispy; **3** Drizzle with pomegranate molasses before serving.

TIPS: **1** Garnish with pomegranate seeds for extra crunch; **2** Serve as a side dish with grilled chicken or fish.

N.V.: Calories: 140, Fat: 7g, Carbs: 17g, Protein: 4g, Sugar: 8g, Sodium: 25 mg, Potassium: 450 mg, Cholesterol: 0 mg, Glucose: 0 mg, Magnesium: 20 mg.

GARLIC HERB STUFFED MUSHROOMS

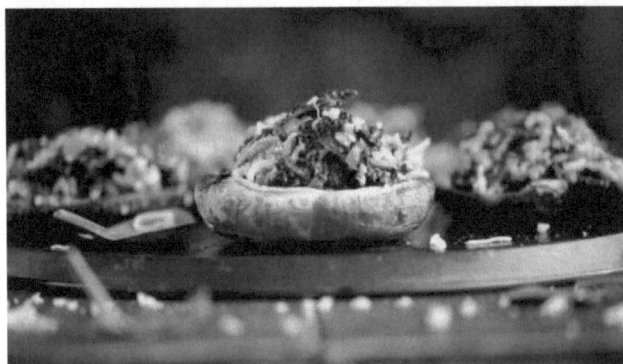

PREPARATION TIME: 15 min **COOKING TIME:** 10 min **MODE OF COOKING:** Baking

INGREDIENTS:

♥12 large mushrooms, stems removed;

♥4 cloves garlic, minced;

♥1/4 cup breadcrumbs;

♥1/4 cup Parmesan cheese, grated;

♥2 Tbsp olive oil;

♥1 Tbsp parsley, chopped

DIRECTIONS: **1** Sauté garlic in olive oil; **2** Mix sautéed garlic with breadcrumbs, Parmesan, and parsley; **3** Stuff mushrooms with the mixture; **4** Bake at 375°F (190°C) until golden.

TIPS: **1** Use gluten-free breadcrumbs for a gluten-sensitive option; **2** Serve warm as an appetizer.

N.V.: Calories: 90, Fat: 6g, Carbs: 7g, Protein: 4g, Sugar: 1g, Sodium: 120 mg, Potassium: 300 mg, Cholesterol: 4 mg, Glucose: 0 mg, Magnesium: 15 mg.

SPICED QUINOA PILAF

PREPARATION TIME: 5 min **COOKING TIME:** 20 min **MODE OF COOKING:** Simmering

INGREDIENTS:

♥1 cup quinoa, rinsed;

♥2 cups vegetable broth;

♥1 tsp cumin;

♥1/2 tsp cinnamon;

♥1/4 cup dried cranberries;

♥1/4 cup almonds, sliced **DIRECTIONS:** **1** Bring quinoa, vegetable broth, cumin, and cinnamon to a boil; **2** Reduce heat and simmer until quinoa is fluffy; **3** Stir in dried cranberries and almonds before serving. **TIPS: 1** Perfect as a hearty side dish; **2** Pair with roasted vegetables. **N.V.:** Calories: 210, Fat: 6g, Carbs: 35g, Protein: 6g, Sugar: 5g, Sodium: 15 mg, Potassium: 240 mg, Cholesterol: 0 mg, Glucose: 0 mg, Magnesium: 70 mg.

BALSAMIC GLAZED SALMON

PREPARATION TIME: 10 min **COOKING TIME:** 15 min **MODE OF COOKING:** Grilling
INGREDIENTS:

- ♥4 salmon fillets, 6 oz each;
- ♥1/4 cup balsamic vinegar;
- ♥1 Tbsp honey;
- ♥1 garlic clove, minced;
- ♥Salt and pepper to taste

DIRECTIONS: 1 Mix balsamic vinegar, honey, and garlic; **2** Season salmon with salt and pepper; **3** Grill salmon, brushing with balsamic glaze until cooked.

TIPS: 1 Serve with a side of steamed asparagus; **2** Ensure the grill is well-oiled to prevent sticking.

N.V.: Calories: 280, Fat: 12g, Carbs: 9g, Protein: 34g, Sugar: 8g, Sodium: 75 mg, Potassium: 800 mg, Cholesterol: 90 mg, Glucose: 0 mg, Magnesium: 50 mg.

SMOKED SALMON AND DILL CROSTINI

PREPARATION TIME: 15 min **COOKING TIME:** 5 min **MODE OF COOKING:** Toasting
INGREDIENTS:

- ♥1 baguette, sliced;
- ♥8 oz smoked salmon;
- ♥1/2 cup cream cheese, softened;
- ♥2 Tbsp fresh dill, chopped;
- ♥1 lemon, juiced

DIRECTIONS: 1 Lightly toast baguette slices; **2** Mix cream cheese with dill and lemon juice; **3** Spread on toast, top with smoked salmon.

TIPS: 1 Capers add a nice tang; **2** Use whole grain baguette for extra fiber.

N.V.: Calories: 180, Fat: 9g, Carbs: 16g, Protein: 12g, Sugar: 2g, Sodium: 560 mg, Potassium: 180 mg, Cholesterol: 20 mg, Glucose: 0 mg, Magnesium: 15 mg.

GRILLED PEACH AND BURRATA SALAD

PREPARATION TIME: 10 min **COOKING TIME:** 6 min **MODE OF COOKING:** Grilling
INGREDIENTS:

♥4 peaches, halved;

♥8 oz burrata cheese;

♥1/4 cup balsamic reduction;

♥1/4 cup basil leaves, torn

DIRECTIONS: 1 Grill peaches cut-side down until charred; **2** Arrange peaches and burrata on a platter; **3** Drizzle with balsamic reduction and sprinkle basil.

TIPS: 1 Add arugula for a peppery bite; **2** Toasted almonds provide a nice crunch.

N.V.: Calories: 290, Fat: 18g, Carbs: 22g, Protein: 13g, Sugar: 16g, Sodium: 40 mg, Potassium: 330 mg, Cholesterol: 40 mg, Glucose: 0 mg, Magnesium: 20 mg.

BEEF TENDERLOIN WITH HERB CRUST

PREPARATION TIME: 20 min **COOKING TIME:** 45 min **MODE OF COOKING:** Roasting

INGREDIENTS:

♥2 lb beef tenderloin;

♥2 Tbsp olive oil;

♥1/4 cup mixed herbs (rosemary, thyme, parsley), chopped;

♥2 cloves garlic, minced;

♥Salt and pepper to taste

DIRECTIONS: 1 Rub tenderloin with olive oil, garlic, herbs, salt, and pepper; **2** Roast at 375°F (190°C) until desired doneness.

TIPS: 1 Let rest before slicing; **2** Serve with a red wine reduction.

N.V.: Calories: 380, Fat: 25g, Carbs: 0g, Protein: 35g, Sugar: 0g, Sodium: 65 mg, Potassium: 500 mg, Cholesterol: 105 mg, Glucose: 0 mg, Magnesium: 40 mg.

PEAR AND ARUGULA SALAD WITH WALNUT VINAIGRETTE

PREPARATION TIME: 10 min **COOKING TIME:** 0 min **MODE OF COOKING:** Mixing

INGREDIENTS:

♥3 pears, sliced;

♥4 cups arugula;

♥1/2 cup walnuts, toasted;

♥1/4 cup walnut oil;

♥2 Tbsp apple cider vinegar;

♥1 tsp honey;

♥Salt and pepper to taste

DIRECTIONS: 1 Whisk walnut oil, vinegar, honey, salt, and pepper for dressing; **2** Toss arugula, pears, and walnuts in dressing.

TIPS: 1 Crumbled goat cheese adds creaminess; **2** Add dried cranberries for a touch of sweetness.

N.V.: Calories: 210, Fat: 15g, Carbs: 19g, Protein: 3g, Sugar: 13g, Sodium: 120 mg, Potassium: 300 mg, Cholesterol: 0 mg, Glucose: 0 mg, Magnesium: 40 mg.

SPINACH AND FETA STUFFED MUSHROOMS

PREPARATION TIME: 15 min **COOKING TIME:** 20 min **MODE OF COOKING:** Baking

INGREDIENTS:

- ♥24 large mushrooms, stems removed;
- ♥1 cup spinach, chopped;
- ♥1/2 cup feta cheese, crumbled;
- ♥1/4 cup breadcrumbs;
- ♥2 Tbsp olive oil;
- ♥2 cloves garlic, minced

DIRECTIONS: 1 Sauté spinach and garlic in olive oil; **2** Mix sautéed spinach, feta, and breadcrumbs; **3** Stuff mixture into mushroom caps; **4** Bake at 350°F (177°C) until mushrooms are tender.

TIPS: 1 Drizzle with balsamic glaze before serving; **2** Add pine nuts for texture.

N.V.: Calories: 70, Fat: 4g, Carbs: 6g, Protein: 3g, Sugar: 2g, Sodium: 180 mg, Potassium: 220 mg, Cholesterol: 5 mg, Glucose: 0 mg, Magnesium: 15 mg.

LEMON HERB ROASTED CHICKEN

PREPARATION TIME: 15 min **COOKING TIME:** 1 hr **MODE OF COOKING:** Roasting

INGREDIENTS:

- ♥1 whole chicken (about 4 lb);
- ♥1 lemon, halved;
- ♥1/4 cup olive oil;
- ♥1/4 cup fresh herbs (thyme, rosemary), chopped;
- ♥3 cloves garlic, minced;
- ♥Salt and pepper to taste

DIRECTIONS: 1 Rub chicken with olive oil, herbs, garlic, salt, and pepper; **2** Stuff with lemon halves; **3** Roast at 400°F (204°C) until juices run clear.

TIPS: 1 Baste with pan juices halfway through; **2** Serve with roasted vegetables.

N.V.: Calories: 410, Fat: 29g, Carbs: 1g, Protein: 35g, Sugar: 0g, Sodium: 85 mg, Potassium: 310 mg, Cholesterol: 105 mg, Glucose: 0 mg, Magnesium: 25 mg.

HERBED QUINOA PILAF WITH ALMONDS

PREPARATION TIME: 10 min **COOKING TIME:** 20 min **MODE OF COOKING:** Simmering

INGREDIENTS:

- ♥1 cup quinoa;
- ♥2 cups vegetable broth;
- ♥1/4 cup sliced almonds;
- ♥1/4 cup fresh parsley, chopped;
- ♥1/4 cup fresh chives, chopped;
- ♥2 Tbsp olive oil;
- ♥Salt and pepper to taste

DIRECTIONS: **1** Rinse quinoa under cold water; **2** Cook quinoa in vegetable broth until liquid is absorbed; **3** Stir in olive oil, almonds, parsley, and chives.

TIPS: **1** Toast the almonds lightly for extra flavor; **2** Serve as a side dish or a light main course.

N.V.: Calories: 220, Fat: 9g, Carbs: 29g, Protein: 8g, Sugar: 1g, Sodium: 150 mg, Potassium: 250 mg, Cholesterol: 0 mg, Glucose: 0 mg, Magnesium: 100 mg.

CREAMY BUTTERNUT SQUASH SOUP

PREPARATION TIME: 15 min **COOKING TIME:** 30 min **MODE OF COOKING:** Boiling

INGREDIENTS:

- ♥1 butternut squash, peeled and cubed;
- ♥1 onion, chopped;
- ♥4 cups vegetable broth;
- ♥1 cup light cream;
- ♥2 Tbsp olive oil;
- ♥Salt and pepper to taste;
- ♥Nutmeg, a pinch

DIRECTIONS: **1** Sauté onion in olive oil until translucent; **2** Add squash and broth, simmer until squash is tender; **3** Puree in blender, return to pot, stir in cream, season with salt, pepper, and nutmeg.

TIPS: **1** Garnish with a swirl of cream and some toasted pumpkin seeds; **2** Add a pinch of cayenne for a spicy kick.

N.V.: Calories: 180, Fat: 9g, Carbs: 24g, Protein: 3g, Sugar: 6g, Sodium: 300 mg, Potassium: 670 mg, Cholesterol: 20 mg, Glucose: 0 mg, Magnesium: 80 mg.

MAPLE GLAZED SALMON

PREPARATION TIME: 10 min **COOKING TIME:** 15 min **MODE OF COOKING:** Grilling

INGREDIENTS:

- ♥4 salmon fillets (6 oz each);
- ♥1/4 cup maple syrup;
- ♥2 Tbsp soy sauce;
- ♥1 garlic clove, minced;
- ♥Salt and pepper to taste

DIRECTIONS: 1 Combine maple syrup, soy sauce, and garlic; **2** Brush glaze over salmon; **3** Grill over medium heat until cooked through.

TIPS: 1 Baste salmon with extra glaze halfway through cooking; **2** Serve with steamed asparagus.

N.V.: Calories: 295, Fat: 15g, Carbs: 10g, Protein: 30g, Sugar: 7g, Sodium: 330 mg, Potassium: 800 mg, Cholesterol: 85 mg, Glucose: 0 mg, Magnesium: 30 mg.

ROASTED VEGETABLE TART

PREPARATION TIME: 20 min **COOKING TIME:** 35 min **MODE OF COOKING:** Baking

INGREDIENTS:

- ♥1 puff pastry sheet;
- ♥1 cup cherry tomatoes;
- ♥1 zucchini, sliced;
- ♥1 bell pepper, sliced;
- ♥1/2 red onion, sliced;
- ♥1/4 cup goat cheese, crumbled;
- ♥2 Tbsp olive oil;
- ♥Salt and pepper to taste

DIRECTIONS: 1 Roll out puff pastry into a tart pan; **2** Arrange vegetables on pastry, drizzle with olive oil, season; **3** Bake at 375°F (190°C) until vegetables are roasted and pastry is golden; **4** Sprinkle with goat cheese before serving.

TIPS: 1 Brush pastry with an egg wash for a glossy finish; **2** Add fresh herbs like thyme or basil after baking for freshness.

N.V.: Calories: 250, Fat: 15g, Carbs: 23g, Protein: 6g, Sugar: 5g, Sodium: 200 mg, Potassium: 300 mg, Cholesterol: 5 mg, Glucose: 0 mg, Magnesium: 25 mg.

MEDITERRANEAN STUFFED PEPPERS

PREPARATION TIME: 20 min **COOKING TIME:** 30 min **MODE OF COOKING:** Baking

INGREDIENTS:

- ♥4 bell peppers, halved and seeded;
- ♥1 cup cooked quinoa;
- ♥1/2 cup feta cheese, crumbled;
- ♥1/2 cup tomatoes, chopped;
- ♥1/4 cup olives, sliced;
- ♥1/4 cup parsley, chopped;
- ♥2 Tbsp olive oil;
- ♥1 lemon, juiced;
- ♥Salt and pepper to taste

DIRECTIONS: **1** Mix quinoa, feta, tomatoes, olives, parsley, lemon juice, and olive oil; **2** Stuff mixture into bell peppers; **3** Bake at 375°F (190°C) until peppers are tender.

TIPS: **1** Serve with a drizzle of tzatziki sauce; **2** Add pine nuts for extra crunch.

N.V.: Calories: 220, Fat: 11g, Carbs: 26g, Protein: 6g, Sugar: 7g, Sodium: 320 mg, Potassium: 350 mg, Cholesterol: 15 mg, Glucose: 0 mg, Magnesium: 40 mg.

FIG AND PROSCIUTTO PIZZA

PREPARATION TIME: 15 min **COOKING TIME:** 10 min **MODE OF COOKING:** Baking

INGREDIENTS:

- ♥1 prebaked pizza crust;
- ♥1/2 cup fig jam;
- ♥6 slices prosciutto;
- ♥1/4 cup arugula;
- ♥1/2 cup mozzarella, shredded;
- ♥1/4 cup balsamic reduction

DIRECTIONS: **1** Spread fig jam on pizza crust; **2** Top with mozzarella and prosciutto; **3** Bake at 450°F (232°C) until cheese melts; **4** Top with arugula and drizzle with balsamic reduction before serving.

TIPS: **1** Fresh fig slices can substitute for jam in season; **2** Garnish with shaved Parmesan.

N.V.: Calories: 290, Fat: 12g, Carbs: 32g, Protein: 12g, Sugar: 15g, Sodium: 560 mg, Potassium: 150 mg, Cholesterol: 25 mg, Glucose: 0 mg, Magnesium: 20 mg.

GRILLED ASPARAGUS WITH LEMON AIOLI

PREPARATION TIME: 10 min **COOKING TIME:** 8 min **MODE OF COOKING:** Grilling

INGREDIENTS:

- ♥1 lb asparagus, trimmed;
- ♥2 Tbsp olive oil;
- ♥Salt and pepper to taste;
- ♥1/2 cup mayonnaise;
- ♥1 garlic clove, minced;
- ♥1 lemon, zested and juiced

DIRECTIONS: 1 Toss asparagus with olive oil, salt, and pepper; **2** Grill until tender; **3** Mix mayonnaise, garlic, lemon zest, and juice to make aioli; **4** Serve asparagus with aioli.

TIPS: 1 Aioli can be prepared ahead and refrigerated; **2** Add parmesan shavings for extra flavor.

N.V.: Calories: 160, Fat: 14g, Carbs: 6g, Protein: 3g, Sugar: 2g, Sodium: 120 mg, Potassium: 250 mg, Cholesterol: 10 mg, Glucose: 0 mg, Magnesium: 20 mg.

LENTIL WALNUT BURGERS

PREPARATION TIME: 20 min **COOKING TIME:** 10 min **MODE OF COOKING:** Pan-frying

INGREDIENTS:

- ♥1 cup cooked lentils;
- ♥1/2 cup walnuts, finely chopped;
- ♥1/4 cup whole wheat breadcrumbs;
- ♥1 egg;
- ♥2 Tbsp parsley, chopped;
- ♥1 garlic clove, minced;
- ♥1 tsp olive oil;
- ♥Salt and pepper to taste

DIRECTIONS: 1 Mash lentils in a bowl; **2** Mix in walnuts, breadcrumbs, egg, parsley, and garlic; **3** Form into patties; **4** Heat olive oil in a pan and cook patties until golden on each side.

TIPS: 1 Serve with a yogurt-based sauce; **2** Great for making in advance and freezing for later use.

N.V.: Calories: 190, Fat: 9g, Carbs: 20g, Protein: 9g, Sugar: 1g, Sodium: 120 mg, Potassium: 340 mg, Cholesterol: 40 mg, Glucose: 0 mg, Magnesium: 50 mg.

SPINACH AND STRAWBERRY SALAD

PREPARATION TIME: 10 min **COOKING TIME:** 0 min **MODE OF COOKING:** Tossing

INGREDIENTS:

- ♥4 cups fresh spinach;
- ♥1 cup strawberries, sliced;
- ♥1/4 cup almonds, sliced;
- ♥2 Tbsp balsamic vinegar;
- ♥1 Tbsp olive oil;
- ♥1 tsp honey;
- ♥Salt and pepper to taste

DIRECTIONS: 1 Combine spinach, strawberries, and almonds in a large bowl; **2** Whisk together vinegar, oil, honey, salt, and pepper; **3** Drizzle dressing over salad and toss gently.

TIPS: 1 Add grilled chicken or fish for extra protein; **2** Perfect for spring and summer gatherings.

N.V.: Calories: 150, Fat: 9g, Carbs: 15g, Protein: 4g, Sugar: 7g, Sodium: 30 mg, Potassium: 380 mg, Cholesterol: 0 mg, Glucose: 0 mg, Magnesium: 60 mg.

ROASTED RED PEPPER AND TOMATO SOUP

PREPARATION TIME: 10 min **COOKING TIME:** 30 min **MODE OF COOKING:** Roasting and Blending

INGREDIENTS:

♥4 red bell peppers, halved and seeded;

♥4 tomatoes, halved;

♥1 onion, chopped;

♥2 cloves garlic;

♥4 cups vegetable broth;

♥1 tsp thyme;

♥1 Tbsp olive oil;

♥Salt and pepper to taste

DIRECTIONS: 1 Place peppers, tomatoes, onion, and garlic on a baking sheet, drizzle with oil, roast at 400°F (204°C) until tender; **2** Blend roasted vegetables with broth and thyme until smooth; **3** Heat soup and season.

TIPS: 1 Serve with a dollop of low-fat Greek yogurt; **2** Roast a head of cauliflower along with peppers for a creamier texture.

N.V.: Calories: 120, Fat: 5g, Carbs: 18g, Protein: 3g, Sugar: 10g, Sodium: 180 mg, Potassium: 500 mg, Cholesterol: 0 mg, Glucose: 0 mg, Magnesium: 30 mg.

GRILLED TURKEY AND VEGETABLE KEBABS

PREPARATION TIME: 15 min **COOKING TIME:** 10 min **MODE OF COOKING:** Grilling

INGREDIENTS:

♥1 lb turkey breast, cut into cubes;

♥1 zucchini, sliced;

♥1 bell pepper, cut into pieces;

♥1 onion, cut into wedges;

♥2 Tbsp olive oil;

♥1 lemon, juiced;

♥2 tsp dried oregano;

♥Salt and pepper to taste

DIRECTIONS: 1 Marinate turkey and vegetables in olive oil, lemon juice, oregano, salt, and pepper for at least 30 min; **2** Thread turkey and vegetables onto skewers; **3** Grill over medium heat until turkey is cooked through.

TIPS: 1 Serve with a side of whole-grain rice or quinoa; **2** Perfect for a healthy BBQ option.

N.V.: Calories: 220, Fat: 7g, Carbs: 10g, Protein: 30g, Sugar: 4g, Sodium: 85 mg, Potassium: 560 mg, Cholesterol: 70 mg, Glucose: 0 mg, Magnesium: 40 mg.

11. 14-Day DASH Diet Meal Plan

Embarking on the DASH Diet's 14-Day Meal Plan is not just about altering what you eat—it's about transforming how you think about meals and your overall approach to health. Over the next two weeks, you'll experience firsthand how a carefully crafted diet can enhance your well-being, boost your energy, and refine your palate to appreciate the subtle, natural flavors of well-prepared food.

This chapter is your stepping stone into a world where food is not seen merely as sustenance, but as a source of life and vitality. The 14-Day Meal Plan has been meticulously designed to ease you into the DASH diet, known for its effectiveness in lowering blood pressure and promoting heart health, but also for its simplicity and approachability. Each day is laid out to provide you with balanced meals that are not only nourishing but also delightful to eat. From breakfast to dinner, including snacks, you'll discover how diverse and flavorful low-sodium cooking can be.

Imagine beginning your day with a breakfast that energizes without weighing you down, enjoying lunches that reinvigorate rather than induce lethargy, and ending with dinners that satisfy both the palate and the body's needs for nutrition. This plan isn't just about feeding the body; it's designed to teach you habits that you can carry beyond these two weeks, integrating them into a sustainable, healthful lifestyle.

Each recipe and meal suggestion comes with complete nutritional information and preparation tips to ensure that even those new to cooking or the DASH diet can follow along easily. You'll also find each day equipped with smart swaps and tips on how to handle cravings, dine out without straying from your goals, and adjust portions to meet your specific needs.

As we move through this meal plan together, think of each meal as a step on the path toward a healthier life. This isn't a temporary diet—it's a way to permanently enhance your relationship with food. Let's enjoy this journey of discovery together, where each meal enriches not just our bodies, but also our lives.

COMPREHENSIVE 14-DAY MENU

WEEK 1	breakfast	snack	lunch	snack	dinner
Monday	Spinach and Feta Omelet	Banana Almond Smoothie	Turkey and Spinach Scrambled	Apple Cinnamon Quinoa Bowl	Tofu and Vegetable Stir-Fry
Tuesday	Blueberry Oatmeal	Greek Yogurt Parfait	Sweet Potato Hash with Eggs	Raspberry Chia Overnight	Peanut Butter Banana Oat
Wednesday	Avocado Toast with Poached Egg	Chia Seed Pudding	Quinoa and Berry Breakfast	Spiced Pumpkin Pancakes	Mediterranean Vegetable Frittata
Thursday	Banana Almond Smoothie	Spinach and Feta Omelet	Apple Cinnamon Quinoa Bowl	Greek Yogurt Parfait	Raspberry Chia Overnight
Friday	Tofu and Vegetable Stir-Fry	Blueberry Oatmeal	Turkey and Spinach Scrambled	Peanut Butter Banana Oat	Spiced Pumpkin Pancakes
Saturday	Quinoa and Berry Breakfast	Chia Seed Pudding	Avocado Toast with Poached Egg	Sweet Potato Hash with Eggs	Mediterranean Vegetable Frittata
Sunday	Greek Yogurt Parfait	Apple Cinnamon Quinoa Bowl	Spinach and Feta Omelet	Blueberry Oatmeal	Tofu and Vegetable Stir-Fry

WEEK 2	breakfast	snack	lunch	snack	dinner
Monday	Quinoa and Berry Breakfast	Greek Yogurt Parfait	Spinach and Feta Omelet	Apple Cinnamon Quinoa Bowl	Tofu and Vegetable Stir-Fry
Tuesday	Blueberry Oatmeal	Chia Seed Pudding	Turkey and Spinach Scrambled	Raspberry Chia Overnight	Peanut Butter Banana Oat
Wednesday	Avocado Toast with Poached Egg	Banana Almond Smoothie	Sweet Potato Hash with Eggs	Spiced Pumpkin Pancakes	Mediterranean Vegetable Frittata
Thursday	Spinach and Feta Omelet	Blueberry Oatmeal	Apple Cinnamon Quinoa Bowl	Greek Yogurt Parfait	Raspberry Chia Overnight
Friday	Tofu and Vegetable Stir-Fry	Quinoa and Berry Breakfast	Turkey and Spinach Scrambled	Peanut Butter Banana Oat	Spiced Pumpkin Pancakes
Saturday	Greek Yogurt Parfait	Chia Seed Pudding	Avocado Toast with Poached Egg	Sweet Potato Hash with Eggs	Mediterranean Vegetable Frittata
Sunday	Apple Cinnamon Quinoa Bowl	Banana Almond Smoothie	Spinach and Feta Omelet	Blueberry Oatmeal	Tofu and Vegetable Stir-Fry

Shopping Lists and Preparation Tips

Embarking on the 14-Day DASH Diet Meal Plan is like setting out on a culinary journey with a map in hand. This map doesn't just guide you from one meal to the next; it teaches you how to shop smartly and prepare meals efficiently, ensuring your success on the diet and beyond. The essence of this journey lies not only in following the meal plan but in embracing the habits that make this diet sustainable and enjoyable.

When you first decide to adopt the DASH diet, the grocery store can feel like a labyrinth. Every aisle holds choices that contribute either positively or negatively to your health goals. The key to navigating this maze is not just knowing what to buy but understanding how to use these ingredients to create meals that are both nourishing and satisfying.

Embrace the Perimeter

Start by rethinking how you navigate the grocery store. The perimeter of the store often houses the freshest ingredients—produce, dairy, and proteins—essential for the DASH diet. These sections should be your primary focus. Here, you'll find the colorful array of fruits and vegetables, lean meats, and low-fat dairy products that form the backbone of your meal plan. Shopping along the store's edges encourages you to load your cart with whole foods, minimizing the temptation from the processed snacks and sweets found in the central aisles.

The Art of Produce Selection

Choosing produce can be an art form. Look for fruits and vegetables that are in season; they are not only more affordable but also at their peak in flavor and nutrition. Vegetables like spinach, kale, and bell peppers, and fruits like berries, apples, and oranges offer a tapestry of flavors and are packed with the vitamins and minerals that the DASH diet celebrates.

When selecting produce, consider variety and color. Each color represents different nutrients and benefits, so a colorful shopping basket means a more diverse intake of vitamins and minerals. For instance, the deep reds of tomatoes and the vibrant oranges of carrots are rich in antioxidants, which are crucial for reducing inflammation and improving heart health.

Proteins: Lean and Mean

When it comes to proteins, opt for lean meats like chicken, turkey, and fish. These provide essential proteins without the high saturated fat content found in many red meats. Fish, such as salmon and mackerel, are rich in omega-3 fatty acids, which are beneficial for heart health. Incorporating plant-based proteins like beans, lentils, and tofu can also add diversity to your meals, providing fiber and reducing your intake of animal fats.

Whole Grains: The Heartier Choice

Don't forget to include whole grains. Whole wheat bread, brown rice, quinoa, and oats are staples under the DASH diet. They provide the necessary fiber to keep your digestive system healthy and help manage blood sugar levels. Choosing whole grains over refined grains ensures that you benefit from the full spectrum of their nutrients without unnecessary additives or sugars.

Dairy: Going Low

In the dairy aisle, focus on low-fat or fat-free options. These provide the calcium and vitamin D necessary for strong bones without the extra fat content of their full-fat counterparts. Yogurt, milk, and cheese can be excellent sources of calcium, but always check labels to ensure there isn't added sugar, which can counteract the benefits of these dairy products.

Preparation: Setting the Stage

Once your shopping is complete, the next step is preparation. A successful implementation of the DASH diet is as much about meal preparation as it is about meal planning. Begin by setting aside time each week to prepare meals. This doesn't mean you need to cook everything in one day but consider washing and chopping vegetables, cooking a batch of whole grains, and portioning out your proteins. This way, when it comes time to cook, much of the work is already done.

Building a Flavor Arsenal

Creating a DASH-friendly kitchen also means having a variety of spices and herbs at your disposal. Since the diet emphasizes low sodium intake, herbs and spices will be your best friends. They add complexity and richness to your meals without the health risks posed by excessive salt use. Experiment with combinations like garlic and rosemary for meats, or cilantro and lime for a zesty touch to salads.

The Role of Healthy Fats

Do not shy away from healthy fats; they are crucial for absorbing vitamins and providing energy. Avocado, nuts, seeds, and olive oil can transform a dish, adding both flavor and texture. For example, a drizzle of olive oil on a salad or some avocado sliced into a wrap can elevate a simple meal while keeping it within the DASH guidelines.

Smart Storage

Finally, consider the storage of your food. Fresh produce can spoil quickly if not stored properly. Investing in good quality storage containers can extend the freshness of your fruits and vegetables, making it easier to stick to your meal plan without frequent trips to the grocery store.

By understanding these principles—shopping wisely, preparing efficiently, and storing correctly—you equip yourself with the tools necessary for success on the DASH diet. Each meal you create will not only bring you closer to achieving your health goals but will also instill lasting habits that extend beyond the 14 days, embedding a healthy rhythm into your lifestyle for years to come.

Shopping list of the week 1

Produce

- ♡ **Spinach**: 3 cups fresh
- ♡ **Bananas**: 3
- ♡ **Apples**: 2
- ♡ **Blueberries**: 1 cup fresh
- ♡ **Avocados**: 4
- ♡ **Sweet potatoes**: 4 medium
- ♡ **Bell peppers**: 2 (mixed colors)
- ♡ **Onions**: 2
- ♡ **Garlic cloves**: 6
- ♡ **Lemons**: 3
- ♡ **Raspberries**: 1/2 cup
- ♡ **Cherry tomatoes**: 1 cup
- ♡ **Arugula**: 4 cups
- ♡ **Broccoli florets**: 1 cup

Proteins

- ♡ **Eggs**: 24 (for various dishes)
- ♡ **Turkey breast**: 1/4 lb cooked
- ♡ **Tofu**: 1/2 lb firm
- ♡ **Chicken breasts**: 4
- ♡ **Salmon fillets**: 4 (4 oz each)

Dairy and Alternatives

- ♡ **Feta cheese**: 1/2 cup crumbled
- ♡ **Greek yogurt**: 3 cups
- ♡ **Low-fat cottage cheese**: 1 cup
- ♡ **Goat cheese**: 3/4 cup crumbled
- ♡ **Parmesan cheese**: 1/2 cup grated
- ♡ **Milk and almond milk**: 2 liters each
- ♡ **Butter**: 1 small pack

Grains and Bakery

- ♡ **Quinoa**: 1 cup
- ♡ **Whole-grain bread**: 8 slices
- ♡ **Rolled oats**: 1 cup
- ♡ **Whole wheat wraps**: 4
- ♡ **Whole wheat pasta**: 2 cups
- ♡ **Whole grain tortillas**: 4

Canned and Jarred Goods

- ♡ **Tuna in water**: 1 can
- ♡ **Chickpeas**: 1 can
- ♡ **Black beans**: 1 can
- ♡ **Coconut milk**: 1 can

Nuts, Seeds, and Dried Fruits

- ♡ **Almond butter**: 2 tbsp
- ♡ **Almonds**: 1/4 cup sliced, 1 tbsp whole
- ♡ **Walnuts**: 1/4 cup chopped
- ♡ **Chia seeds**: 5 tbsp
- ♡ **Pine nuts**: 1/4 cup

Spices and Seasonings

- ♡ **Olive oil**: 500 ml
- ♡ **Vinegar (white and balsamic)**: 100 ml each
- ♡ **Salt and pepper**: as needed
- ♡ **Cinnamon**: 1 tsp
- ♡ **Nutmeg**: 1/4 tsp
- ♡ **Smoked paprika**: 1/2 tsp
- ♡ **Cumin**: 1 tsp
- ♡ **Chili powder**: 1/2 tsp
- ♡ **Fresh herbs (dill, parsley)**: 1 bunch each
- ♡ **Sesame seeds**: 2 tbsp

♡ **Ginger**: 1 small root

Condiments and Sauces

♡ **Mayonnaise**: 100 ml

♡ **Sriracha sauce**: 1 tsp

♡ **Caesar dressing**: 1/2 cup

♡ **Soy sauce**: 1/4 cup

♡ **Sesame oil**: 1 tbsp

♡ **Maple syrup**: 3 tbsp

♡ **Honey**: 4 tbsp

♡ **Pesto**: 1/2 cup

♡ **Cranberry sauce**: 1/4 cup

Snacks and Misc

♡ **Granola**: 1/4 cup

♡ **Vanilla extract**: 1/2 tsp

♡ **Coconut flakes**: a handful

Shopping list of the week 2

Produce

♡ **Spinach**: 3 cups fresh

♡ **Bananas**: 3

♡ **Apples**: 2

♡ **Blueberries**: 1 cup fresh

♡ **Avocados**: 4

♡ **Sweet potatoes**: 4 medium

♡ **Bell peppers**: 2 (mixed colors)

♡ **Onions**: 2

♡ **Garlic cloves**: 6

♡ **Lemons**: 3

♡ **Raspberries**: 1/2 cup

♡ **Cherry tomatoes**: 1 cup

♡ **Arugula**: 4 cups

♡ **Broccoli florets**: 1 cup

Proteins

♡ **Eggs**: 24 (for various dishes)

♡ **Turkey breast**: 1/4 lb cooked

♡ **Tofu**: 1/2 lb firm

♡ **Chicken breasts**: 4

♡ **Salmon fillets**: 4 (4 oz each)

Dairy and Alternatives

♡ **Feta cheese**: 1/2 cup crumbled

♡ **Greek yogurt**: 3 cups

♡ **Low-fat cottage cheese**: 1 cup

♡ **Goat cheese**: 3/4 cup crumbled

♡ **Parmesan cheese**: 1/2 cup grated

♡ **Milk and almond milk**: 2 liters each

♡ **Butter**: 1 small pack

Grains and Bakery

♡ **Quinoa**: 1 cup

♡ **Whole-grain bread**: 8 slices

♡ **Rolled oats**: 1 cup

♡ **Whole wheat wraps**: 4

♡ **Whole wheat pasta**: 2 cups

♡ **Whole grain tortillas**: 4

Canned and Jarred Goods

♡ **Tuna in water**: 1 can

♡ **Chickpeas**: 1 can

♡ **Black beans**: 1 can

♡ **Coconut milk**: 1 can

Nuts, Seeds, and Dried Fruits

♡ **Almond butter**: 2 tbsp

♡ **Almonds**: 1/4 cup sliced, 1 tbsp whole

♡ **Walnuts**: 1/4 cup chopped

♡ **Chia seeds**: 5 tbsp

♡ **Pine nuts**: 1/4 cup

Spices and Seasonings

- ♡ **Olive oil**: 500 ml
- ♡ **Vinegar (white and balsamic)**: 100 ml each
- ♡ **Salt and pepper**: as needed
- ♡ **Cinnamon**: 1 tsp
- ♡ **Nutmeg**: 1/4 tsp
- ♡ **Smoked paprika**: 1/2 tsp
- ♡ **Cumin**: 1 tsp
- ♡ **Chili powder**: 1/2 tsp
- ♡ **Fresh herbs (dill, parsley)**: 1 bunch each
- ♡ **Sesame seeds**: 2 tbsp
- ♡ **Ginger**: 1 small root

Condiments and Sauces

- ♡ **Mayonnaise**: 100 ml
- ♡ **Sriracha sauce**: 1 tsp
- ♡ **Caesar dressing**: 1/2 cup
- ♡ **Soy sauce**: 1/4 cup
- ♡ **Sesame oil**: 1 tbsp
- ♡ **Maple syrup**: 3 tbsp
- ♡ **Honey**: 4 tbsp
- ♡ **Pesto**: 1/2 cup
- ♡ **Cranberry sauce**: 1/4 cup

Snacks and Misc

- ♡ **Granola**: 1/4 cup
- ♡ **Vanilla extract**: 1/2 tsp
- ♡ **Coconut flakes**: a handful

12. Beyond the Book: Maintaining a Healthy Lifestyle

As you turn the pages of this guide and incorporate its principles into your daily life, you begin to see that maintaining a healthy lifestyle extends far beyond the confines of any book. It's about embedding these new habits into every facet of your day, ensuring that each choice contributes to a sustained sense of well-being. This chapter is designed to help you navigate the ongoing journey of health, long after the last recipe has been tried and the final page turned.

Imagine your life as a garden that you cultivate daily. The seeds you've sown throughout this book—knowledge of nutritious foods, understanding of balanced meals, and insights into effective meal planning—are just the beginning. Like any garden, the beauty and bounty come not just from planting but from consistent care. This ongoing cultivation requires patience, adaptability, and a commitment to continual growth and learning.

Living a healthy lifestyle means more than just eating well when it's convenient; it's about making thoughtful choices that align with your long-term goals. It's about finding joy in the preparation of a meal, relishing the crunch of fresh vegetables, and savoring the richness of whole grains. Each meal is an opportunity to nourish not just your body, but also your mind and soul.

However, the path isn't always clear or easy. There will be obstacles—unexpected life changes, holidays, and social gatherings—that might seem like barriers to your goals. Yet, it's precisely these challenges that test your commitment and allow you to flex your newfound knowledge. This chapter offers strategies to enhance your resilience, ensuring that you can maintain balance and health through life's ups and downs, making healthy living not just a phase but a permanent and fulfilling aspect of your life.

By embracing the lessons of this book and continuing to apply them every day, you ensure that your journey towards health is vibrant and enduring. Let's explore how to keep the momentum going, integrating the principles of the DASH diet into a lifestyle that's as rewarding as it is wholesome.

Long-Term Strategies for Success

Maintaining a healthy lifestyle is akin to steering a ship on an open sea. The initial thrill of setting sail on calm waters—the excitement of starting a new diet or health regimen—eventually meets the unpredictable tides of everyday life. The long-term success of navigating these waters doesn't lie just in the strength of the initial push; it depends profoundly on your ability to adjust the sails, to redirect and maintain course through both calm and stormy weather. This section delves into the strategies that will help you sustain and thrive in your commitment to a healthy lifestyle, embedding the principles of the DASH diet into your daily rhythm permanently.

Adaptability: Your Greatest Ally

Life is fluid, ever-changing, and the ability to adapt is crucial. A rigid diet plan that doesn't bend with the circumstances of your life is likely to break. Instead, fostering adaptability involves understanding the core principles of the DASH diet—low sodium, high fiber, and balanced nutrients—and applying them in flexible ways. For example, if you find yourself at a restaurant or a friend's dinner party, choose dishes that emphasize vegetables and lean proteins, and don't be shy about asking for dressings or sauces on the side to control sodium intake.

Education: An Ongoing Journey

Knowledge is the wind in your sails; it propels you forward and keeps you moving in the right direction. Continuing to educate yourself about nutritional science and health can reinforce your commitment and interest in your diet. This might mean subscribing to health and wellness magazines, following reputable health food blogs, or joining community groups that focus on healthy living. The more you understand the reasons behind the DASH principles, the more motivated you will be to stick to them, knowing they are backed by solid science.

Mindfulness: The Art of Conscious Eating

Mindfulness, or the practice of being present and fully engaged with the task at hand, can transform the way you eat. It's about more than just slowing down or enjoying your food—it's about listening to your body and responding to its cues. Are you really hungry, or just bored? Does your body feel better with less sugar, more fiber, or a heavier lean protein intake? Being mindful about your eating involves creating meals thoughtfully, eating without distractions like the TV or smartphone, and noticing how food affects your mood and physical state.

Routine: The Framework of Success

While flexibility is crucial, so too is a solid routine. Humans are creatures of habit, and establishing a set routine for meal planning, shopping, and preparation can reduce the mental load of making healthy choices. Dedicate time each week to plan your meals, shop for ingredients, and prepare what you can in advance. This not only helps to alleviate stress but ensures that you have healthy options on hand when you're too tired to cook or tempted to stray from your goals.

Community: Finding Strength in Numbers

You're not in this alone. Engaging with a community that shares your health goals can provide a significant boost to your motivation. Whether it's a local cooking class, an online forum, or a group exercise class, being part of a community can offer support, inspire new ideas, and give you a sense of accountability. Sharing your journey, challenges, and successes with others can also help to normalize the lifestyle changes you are making and integrate them more fully into your everyday life.

Resilience: Bouncing Back with Grace

Setbacks are a natural part of any journey, and the path to maintaining a healthy lifestyle is no different. The key to resilience is not in avoiding these setbacks but in how you respond to them. If you indulge in a high-sodium meal or skip a few days of balanced eating, don't let this derail your entire plan. Acknowledge the slip, learn from it, and then get right back on track. The ability to rebound strengthens your commitment and teaches you valuable lessons about what triggers your detours.

Self-compassion: The Soothing Balm

Be kind to yourself. Change is hard, and self-criticism can be demotivating. Practice self-compassion by recognizing that perfection is unattainable and that each small step you take is part of a larger journey toward health. Celebrate your victories, no matter how small, and treat yourself with the same kindness and encouragement you would offer a good friend.

Personalization: Your Unique Path

Finally, remember that the DASH diet, like any diet, is not one-size-fits-all. Personalize your approach by paying attention to how foods make you feel, consulting with healthcare providers, and adjusting your diet to fit your specific health needs and taste preferences. This personalized approach not only makes the diet more effective but also more enjoyable and sustainable in the long term.

By weaving these strategies into the fabric of your daily life, you craft a lifestyle that supports not just your physical health but also your mental and emotional well-being. This holistic approach ensures that your journey on the DASH diet is not just a fleeting endeavor but a lasting, enriching experience that continues

ADDITIONAL RESOURCES AND SUPPORT

Embarking on a journey toward a healthier lifestyle with the DASH diet at your side is like setting out on a voyage of discovery—a quest to better understand not only your dietary needs but your body's overall health. Along the way, the guidance from a comprehensive array of resources and the support from communities can act like beacons and anchors, providing light and stability as you navigate this new territory. This section is dedicated to outlining the additional resources and support systems that can enrich your journey, ensuring you're never truly going it alone.

The Power of Continuing Education

Education is a lifelong process, particularly when it comes to health and wellness. As nutritional science evolves, staying informed through credible sources is vital. Books, peer-reviewed journals, and educational websites can be invaluable resources. Consider subscribing to newsletters from institutions like the American Heart Association or the Mayo Clinic, which regularly publish updates on heart health and nutrition that are directly applicable to the DASH diet principles.

Harnessing Digital Tools

In the digital age, numerous apps and websites offer practical assistance in tracking your dietary habits, physical activity, and overall progress. Apps such as MyFitnessPal or Fat Secret allow you to monitor your food intake and exercise, adjusting easily to your specific needs on the DASH diet. These tools can help you maintain accountability and provide insights into your nutritional patterns, making it easier to stay on track.

Building a Support Network

Support can also come from online forums and local community groups focusing on health, nutrition, and wellness. Participating in discussions and sharing experiences can provide motivational support and deepen your understanding of the practical aspects of maintaining a healthy lifestyle. Websites like SparkPeople or in-person meetup groups offer platforms where encouragement and advice flow freely, helping to sustain your commitment in the long term.

Professional Guidance

For personalized advice, consulting with healthcare professionals such as dietitians, nutritionists, and your primary healthcare provider is crucial. These experts can offer tailored guidance based on your health status, dietary needs, and any medical conditions. Regular check-ups and consultations can help adjust your diet plan to better suit your changing health needs, providing a level of customization that goes beyond general guidelines.

Educational Workshops and Cooking Classes

Learning can be more engaging and enjoyable when it's hands-on. Look for cooking classes and nutritional workshops in your area that focus on low-sodium cooking techniques, the principles of the DASH diet, or general healthy eating strategies. These classes not only enhance your cooking skills but also expand your repertoire of recipes, making it easier to enjoy a variety of healthy meals without feeling restricted.

Volunteer Opportunities

Engaging with your community through volunteer opportunities can also support your lifestyle changes. Many communities have gardens, farmer's markets, or outreach programs that focus on nutrition and health. These can be wonderful ways to learn more about food sourcing, sustainable eating, and can even offer opportunities to teach others about the benefits of a healthy diet.

Advocacy and Beyond

As you grow more confident and informed about your health choices, consider advocating for healthier food options in your local schools, workplaces, and community centers. Advocacy can be a powerful way to enhance your commitment to your lifestyle changes and can help improve public health at the community level.

Documentaries and Media

Immersing yourself in documentaries and media related to health, diet, and wellness can be another enriching way to support your lifestyle changes. Films and documentaries that explore the science of nutrition, the effects of sodium on health, or stories of personal health transformations can be profoundly motivating and enlightening.

Blogs and Social Media

Following health and wellness influencers who focus on practical, science-backed nutrition advice can also be beneficial. Platforms like Instagram, Pinterest, and personal blogs are full of creative ideas and can be sources of inspiration for meals and healthy lifestyle tips. However, always consider the credibility of the source to ensure the information is reliable and based on sound nutritional science.

By leveraging these resources and tapping into various forms of support, you can enrich your journey toward a healthier lifestyle. Each resource acts not just as a guide but also as a companion and catalyst, propelling you forward with renewed knowledge, skills, and enthusiasm. Your path to wellness is not just about the food you eat—it's about continuously learning, engaging with others, and finding joy in every step of the journey.

ENCOURAGING A LIFETIME OF HEALTHY HABITS

Embarking on a journey toward a healthier lifestyle is akin to planting a garden. It requires patience, care, and consistent effort. The seeds you sow today—the habits you develop and the choices you make—will cultivate a future of wellness and vitality. As you close this book and continue on your path, the principles of the DASH diet can serve as your guide, not just in diet but as a foundation for a life well-lived. This sub-chapter aims to weave the thread of these principles through the fabric of your daily life, encouraging a lifetime of healthy habits.

Integrating Wellness into Daily Routines

To make a lasting impact, wellness should not be viewed as a separate or temporary effort but integrated into your everyday routine. Start with small, manageable changes that do not overwhelm but instead empower you. For instance, begin by incorporating more vegetables into your meals or replacing soda with water throughout the day. Over time, these small changes become part of your lifestyle, almost second nature, gradually building a stronger foundation for more significant changes.

The Power of Morning Rituals

How you start your day often sets the tone for the hours that follow. Establishing a morning ritual can have a profound impact on your overall health. This might involve starting the day with a glass of water to rehydrate, a short walk to invigorate the body, or a few minutes of meditation to clear the mind. These rituals anchor your day, providing clarity and purpose.

Smart Grocery Shopping

Carrying the principles of the DASH diet into your shopping habits ensures that your pantry and refrigerator support your health goals. Make a habit of reading labels, not just for calorie content but for sodium levels, types of fats, and the presence of added sugars. Opt for fresh produce, lean proteins, and whole grains as staples of your diet. By stocking your home with these healthful options, you make maintaining a healthy diet more effortless.

Cultivating the Joy of Cooking

Rediscover the pleasure in preparing your own meals. Cooking at home allows you to control ingredients, methods of preparation, and portion sizes—all crucial for adhering to the DASH diet. Experiment with herbs and spices to enhance flavors without adding salt. Embrace the process of cooking as a therapeutic activity, not just a necessity.

Regular Physical Activity

Regular exercise is a cornerstone of good health, complementing the nutritional aspects of the DASH diet. Find activities you enjoy, be it yoga, cycling, swimming, or simple daily walks. The key is consistency and enjoyment. Exercise should not feel like a chore but rather a rewarding, integral part of your day.

Staying Informed and Educated

Knowledge is a powerful tool in maintaining a healthy lifestyle. Stay informed about the latest research in nutrition and health. Subscribe to health newsletters, listen to podcasts, or read books that expand your understanding of your body and its needs. This ongoing education will not only inspire you but will also empower you to make informed decisions about your health.

Building a Support Network

Surround yourself with a community that supports and shares your health goals. This could be a cooking club, a fitness group, or online communities focused on healthy living. Sharing your challenges and successes with others provides motivation and accountability, which are crucial for long-term adherence to a healthy lifestyle.

Mindfulness and Mental Health

Mental and emotional well-being is just as important as physical health. Practice mindfulness, which can enhance your emotional resilience and reduce stress—a significant factor in overall health. Techniques like deep breathing, mindfulness meditation, or keeping a gratitude journal can improve your mental health and, by extension, your physical health.

Regular Health Check-Ups

Regular visits to your healthcare provider for check-ups can help monitor your health status and catch any potential health issues early. These check-ups provide an opportunity to discuss your diet and lifestyle changes and get professional feedback on your progress.

Celebrate Your Progress

Finally, remember to celebrate your progress, no matter how small. Set goals and reward yourself when you achieve them. These rewards could be a new cookbook, a new outfit, or a new kitchen gadget. Celebrating your successes reinforces your motivation and commitment to a healthy lifestyle.

By embedding these practices into your daily life, you create a sustainable way of living that not only adheres to the DASH diet but also enriches your overall quality of life. This journey is unique for everyone, and these guidelines are meant to be adapted to fit your personal needs, preferences, and lifestyle, ensuring that the healthy habits you form are enjoyable and lasting.

Volume Equivalents (Liquid)

US Standard	US Standard (ounces)	Metric (approximate)
2 tablespoons	1 fl. oz.	30 mL
¼ cup	2 fl. oz.	60 mL
half cup	4 fl. oz.	120 mL
1 cup	8 fl. oz.	240 mL
1 half cups	12 fl. oz.	355 mL
2 cups or 1 pint	16 fl. oz.	457 mL
4 cups or 1 quart	32 fl. oz.	1 L
1 gallon	128 fl. oz.	4 L

Volume Equivalents (Dry)

US Standard	Metric (approximate)
1/8 teaspoon	0.5 mL
¼ teaspoon	1 mL
half teaspoon	2 mL
¾ teaspoon	4 mL
1 teaspoon	5 mL
1 tablespoon	15 mL
¼ cup	59 mL
1/3 cup	79 mL
half cup	118 mL
2/3 cup	156 mL
¾ cup	177 mL
1 cup	235 mL
2 cups or 1 pint	475 mL
3 cups	700 mL
4 cups or 1 quart	1 L

Fahrenheit (F)	Celsius (C) (approximate)
250°F	120°C
300°F	150°C
325°F	165°C
350°F	180°C
375°F	190°C
400°F	200°C
425°F	220°C
450°F	230°C

Weight Equivalents

US Standard	Metric (approximate)
1 tablespoon	15 g
half ounce	15 g
1 ounce	30 g
2 ounces	60 g
4 ounces	115 g
8 ounces	225 g
12 ounces	340 g
16 ounces or 1 pound or 1 lb	455 g

SCAN QR CODE TO ACCESS EXTRA CONTENT

Made in United States
Troutdale, OR
02/25/2025